DATE DUE

835080	5/28/94
4888324	12/24/94
8/4/97	
74/011	MAY 0 3 1998
ALA	MAR 1 2 2000
JUL 31 2002	
GAYLORD	PRINTED IN U.S.A.

Guillain-Barré Syndrome

Gareth J. Parry, M.B., F.R.A.C.P.
Professor of Neurology
University of Minnesota
Minneapolis, Minnesota

With a contribution by

J.D. Pollard, PH.D., B.SC.(MED.), F.R.A.C.P.
Professor of Medicine
University of Sydney
Sydney, Australia

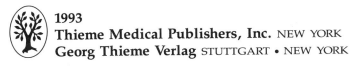

1993
Thieme Medical Publishers, Inc. NEW YORK
Georg Thieme Verlag STUTTGART • NEW YORK

RC
416
.P37
1993

Thieme Medical Publishers, Inc.
381 Park Avenue South
New York, New York 10016

GUILLAIN-BARRÉ SYNDROME
Gareth J. Parry, M.D.

Library of Congress Cataloging-in-Publication Data

Parry, Gareth J.,
    Guillain-Barré Syndrome / Gareth J. Parry; with a contribution by
J.D. Pollard.
      p.   cm.
    Includes bibliographical references and index.
    ISBN 0-86577-444-7—ISBN 3-13-783601-8
    1. Polyradiculoneuritis.   I. Pollard , J. D. (John David)
II. Title.
    [DNLM: 1. Polyradiculoneuritis. WL 544 P264g]
RC416.P37 1993
616.8'7—dc20
DNLM/DLC
for Library of Congress   92-49287
                                                       CIP

Important note: Medicine is an ever-changing science. Research and clinical experience are
continually broadening our knowledge, in particular our knowledge of proper treatment and
drug therapy. Insofar as this book mentions any dosage or applications, readers may rest assured
that the authors, editors, and publishers have made every effort to ensure that such references
are strictly in accordance with the state of knowledge at the time of production of the book.
Nevertheless, every user is requested to carefully examine the manufacturers' leaflets accompanying each drug to check on his own responsibility whether the dosage schedules recommended therein or the contraindications stated by the manufacturers differ from the statements
made in the present book. Such examination is particularly important with drugs that are either
rarely used or have been newly released on the market.

Some of the product names, patents, and registered designs referred to in this book are in fact
registered trademarks or proprietary names even though specific reference to this fact is not
always made in the text. Therefore, the appearance of a name without designation as proprietary
is not to be construed as a representation by the publisher that it is in the public domain.

Printed in the United States of America.

5 4 3 2 1

TMP ISBN 0-86577-444-7
GTV ISBN 3-13-783601-8

Contents

Foreword

It is truly a privilege to be invited to write a foreword to this excellent monograph on Guillain-Barré syndrome and the related chronic inflammatory demyelinating neuropathies. Dr. Gareth Parry and I have been friends and colleagues for many years. We are both graduates of the University of Otago Medical School, in New Zealand, where we were greatly influenced by a neurophysiological tradition established by Sir John Eccles and carried forward by Professor A.K. McIntyre. We were both later influenced by the Peripheral Nerve group established by Dr. Arthur K. Asbury at the University of Pennsylvania. Over the years, we have enjoyed debating many of the concepts advanced in this book, and this has been particularly so in the past four years at the Louisiana State University Medical Center in New Orleans. The review of chronic inflammatory demyelinating polyneuropathy (CIDP) is based predominantly on recent experience at LSU. Be in no doubt, however, that this work is Dr. Parry's alone, and for me it is exciting to see how he has developed and refined many of these ideas.

This monograph places special emphasis on the value of electrophysiology, not only in the diagnosis and prognosis, but also in the elucidation of the pathophysiological basis of these disorders. I share this approach and stress its emphasis. These acquired demyelinating neuropathies are endlessly fascinating to clinical neurophysiologists because they encompass a wide and variable pathophysiology, both in time and space. Although there appear to be favored sites of peripheral nerve lesions—for example, proximal roots, plexi, intramuscular nerve twigs and sites of subclinical entrapment—it is evident that the pattern and severity of lesions is quite variable from patient to patient. Especially in CIDP the sites of focal inflammatory demyelination are responsible for very different clinical presentations. The generalized symmetrical sensorimotor pattern is not invariable and the contrasting clinical features of mononeuritis multiplex, multifocal motor syndrome, or predominantly sensory locomotor ataxia are all encountered. Each patient studied becomes a unique physiological experiment and should be approached as such.

Recent advances in immunology and the nature of the infectious agents known to trigger the acute disease are of course no less important and are well reviewed. The discussion of clinical features, neuropathology, and experience in managing the inflammatory demyelinating neuropathies by intravenous immunoglobulin and other immunotherapies is timely and comprehensive. I can confidently recommend this monograph to neurologists, intensive care specialists, clinical neurophysiologists, internists, physiatrists, and other physicians responsible for the care of patients.

Austin J. Sumner, M.D.

Preface

When work was started on this volume in 1987, it was envisaged as a practical and highly clinical guide to the neophyte in disorders of peripheral nerve. Since that time it has steadily expanded into what I hope is a comprehensive review of the Guillain-Barré syndrome, with a particular emphasis on the electrophysiology of demyelination. I hope that despite this expansion, the book achieves its original purpose while at the same time appealing to a wider audience.

Many individuals have fostered my interest in disorders of peripheral nerve. I would like to acknowledge particularly the important influence of Martin Pollock and Austin J. Sumner. The former, by his example and enthusiasm, steered me toward a career in neurology and stimulated my interest in the peripheral nervous system. The latter encouraged me to take my training at the University of Pennsylvania, rather than follow the example of most of my countrymen who studied in the United Kingdom. During our long friendship and professional association, Dr. Sumner has constantly challenged and stimulated me, making me a better neurologist and a more critical investigator. While at the University of Pennsylvania I was also influenced by Arthur K. Asbury and Mark J. Brown of the Peripheral Nerve Laboratories there, and I was provided with the kind of intellectually rigorous environment that has kept me in the United States. Without the guidance and friendship of these and many other individuals, this book would never have been written and I am grateful to them.

I would also like to acknowledge the contributions of three editors who helped to prepare this book. First, I am grateful to Maria Sarro, formerly of Thieme Medical Publishers, whose encouragement helped to overcome my initial apprehensions about the project, and to Kimberly Wright, also of Thieme, who courteously, but with great persistence, kept my nose to the grindstone so that the manuscript was finished not too far behind schedule. Second, I am indebted to my wife, Catherine Parry, who diplomatically complimented me on my writing at the same time as she mended my fractured syntax, reunited my split infinitives, corrected my spelling, and generally improved the sense of the language, sometimes to the detriment of her own deadlines.

Gareth J. Parry, M.B., F.R.A.C.P.

History of Guillain-Barré Syndrome

In 1916 Guillain, Barré, and Strohl[1] published their now famous account of radiculoneuritis with albuminocytologic dissociation, the condition that now bears their name. However, recognition of this particular clinical entity preceded them by about 80 years and, in retrospect, several hundred cases of an identical disorder had been described in the intervening period.

Clinical Descriptions

The Syndrome of Peripheral Neuritis

Given the frequency with which peripheral neuropathy is diagnosed today, the entity has a remarkably short history. The first clinical account of what was almost certainly peripheral neuropathy was published in 1787 by John Lettsom as a complication of excessive alcohol use.[2] Although he described the clinical features with remarkable vividness and clarity, he made no allusion to the anatomical and pathological basis for the symptoms and signs. Unaware of the earlier graphic report, James Jackson provided an equally vivid clinical description of alcoholic neuropathy 35 years later, in 1822, again without recognizing anatomical or pathological features.[3] In fact, he thought that the disease was localized in skin and muscle. In 1828 in Paris there was a remarkable epidemic of neuropathy that was almost certainly of a toxic nature. Detailed clinical descriptions were published by Auguste-François Chomel and brain and spinal cord from two cases were examined pathologically, but no cause for the condition identified.[4] The English physician, Robert Graves, better known for his descriptions of thyrotoxicosis, also studied the same epidemic, and was the first to suggest that the peripheral nerves were the seat of the disorder but provided no pathological confirmation of his hypothesis.[5] The first confirmation that pathological changes occurred in peripheral nerves did not appear for another 20 years. In 1864, Louis Dumenil of Rouen,[6] fully aware of the earlier suggestion of Graves, examined the peripheral nerves of a 71-year-old man who had died 5 months after the onset of a subacutely progressive, ascending paralysis with distal sensory loss. There was loss of nerve fibers in the distal peripheral nerves of the arms and legs but the proximal nerves to clinically unaffected muscles, nerve roots, and the spinal cord and brain were normal. Two years later, Dumenil described three more cases and coined the term "chronic neuritis."[7] Dumenil is largely responsible for placing the pathological diagnosis of peripheral neuropathy on a firm footing, although many of the most prominent neurologists of that time remained reluctant to accept the concept. For example, the influential French neurologist Vulpian continued to insist that the syndrome of neuritis was a meningomyelitis, more than 15 years after Dumenil's descriptions.[8] However, the concept gained increasing acceptance and many reports of neuritis resulting from diphtheria and lead intoxication and of what was almost certainly the Guillain-Barré syndrome soon followed. The evolution up to the end of the 19th century of our understanding of the concept "neuritis" is well reviewed by Viets.[9]

The Guillain-Barré Syndrome

EARLY DESCRIPTIONS

The first clinical descriptions of what is now known as the Guillain-Barré syndrome probably were those that appeared in the 1830s. In 1834, an English physician, James Wardrop, reported on a case with many clinical features that could hardly have any other cause.[10] A 35-year-old man developed numbness that ascended his left leg before spreading to other limbs and briefly preceded loss of strength. Over the subsequent 10 days he lost all power except for the ability to turn his head and move his toes. Although no comment was made on respirations, they were presumably normal. Despite sensory symptoms, the sensory examination was normal as were bowel, bladder, and vital functions. This paralytic illness was preceded by diarrhea. Upon treatment by purging, the patient began to recover and "several years afterward (he was) in the enjoyment of good health, having never had any return of the symptoms." In 1837, the French neurologist, Ollivier, from Bordeaux, described two patients with acutely evolving paralysis.[11] One patient developed symptoms after normal parturition and died 2 days later. Autopsy failed to reveal any pathological abnormality of the brain or spinal cord but peripheral nerves were not examined. The second patient developed severe weakness of all limbs as well as truncal, respiratory, and cranial innervated muscles and yet made a spontaneous recovery. The recovery of strength in Wardrop's case and in one of Ollivier's was an extraordinary occurrence given the grim prognosis for severe poliomyelitis, the usual acute paralytic illness of the day.

LANDRY'S PARALYSIS

In 1859, Jean-Baptiste Octave Landry published a detailed clinical description of a patient with an acute paralytic illness that evolved over a period of 8 days from the onset of weakness to death.[12] There had been a variety of systemic symptoms over the preceding year and a half and an ill-defined period of acral paresthesiae preceding paralysis. Although the paralysis ascended as the disease progressed, Landry noted that the proximal arm muscles were affected before the distal ones and, even when the paralysis was advanced, some hand movement was preserved when proximal arm movement was completely lost. Muscles of the thorax and abdomen were involved, including the diaphragm, resulting in respiratory difficulty, although it appeared to be mild. There was some weakness of the tongue and jaw and swallowing was impaired. There was no muscular atrophy. Despite profound paralysis, "the electric reactions of the muscles and nerves were normal," consistent with what we now know to be conduction block at proximal sites. Sensation was not as much involved. Initially, perception of pain and temperature had not changed but proprioception was markedly reduced; later there was distal pansensory loss. All reflexes were lost. There was a resting tachycardia, distal extremities were cold despite high seasonal temperature, and sphincter weakness was also noted. Death was sudden and may have been due to arrhythmia since there did not appear to have been significant respiratory compromise, by clinical criteria, at the time of death. Thus, all of the classical clinical features of what is now known as the Guillain-Barré syndrome were clearly manifested and carefully documented by Landry. There were premonitory sensory symptoms and muscle cramps but only minor sensory signs that affected proprioception more than cutaneous sensibility. The alteration in sensation began in the feet and ascended to the legs, thighs, and eventually to the arms. Severe weakness evolved over 8 days. It appeared to begin in the quadriceps; the patient's first complaint was that he "noticed that his knees often gave way while walking" and ascended only in that the legs were involved before the arms. This early involvement of proximal muscles has been repeatedly confirmed and yet the popular misconception of an ascending paralysis, involving distal muscles before the more proximal ones, persists today. Cranial and respiratory muscles were also involved. There was complete areflexia. What we now recognize as autonomic involvement was present, manifested as "sphincter weakness," resting tachycardia, and cold distal extremities, and may have contributed to his death. In addition to this case described in such exquisite detail, Landry noted that he had seen four other cases and had gleaned five more, including those of Ollivier, from the literature of the day. Of these 10 cases, only two were fatal; the remainder recovered, with recovery of function occurring in the reverse order to the loss of function. Landry considered that the trivial "congestion of the membranes" of the brain and spinal cord was insufficient to account for the paralysis but does not appear to have considered peripheral nerves as a potential site for the pathology. Numerous reports of "Landry's paralysis" appeared in the latter half of the 19th century but little was added in the way of clinical features to the original description. In fact, no significant new observations have been added in the clinical arena to the present, except perhaps for the observation of C. Miller Fisher that the syndrome of ophthalmoplegia, ataxia, and areflexia was a form of the Guillain-Barré syndrome.[13]

GUILLAIN, BARRÉ, AND STROHL

The next important contribution to our understanding of this disorder came in 1916, when Guillain, Barré, and Strohl published their now famous observations on "radiculoneuritis with hyperalbuminosis of the cerebrospinal fluid without cellular reaction," which led to the current eponymous designation of the syndrome.[1] They described two soldiers with an acutely evolving, nonfatal, generalized paralysis similar in all respects to the many previous reports. Although Guillain, in particular, vigorously contested any suggestion that their cases represented examples of Landry's paralysis, there are no substantive differences in the clinical features. However, they pointed out for the first time one of the cardinal manifestations of the syndrome, namely, the marked elevation of cerebrospinal fluid (CSF) protein without a concomitant increase in cells. This albuminocytologic dissociation was a well recognized feature of diphtheritic neuropathy[14] but had not, to that point, been described in other disorders of peripheral nerve. In 1917, Queckenstedt independently noted albuminocytologic dissociation in three cases of idiopathic polyneuritis that may also have been examples of the same disorder, although no clinical features of the cases are given.[15] It was primarily the albuminocytologic dissociation that ultimately led Draganescu and Claudian, in 1927, to designate the disorder the "Guillain-Barré syndrome."[16] Andre Strohl was an electrophysiologist who probably contributed the observation that responses of nerves and muscles to electrical stimulation was preserved. It is not entirely clear why Draganescu and Claudian omitted Strohl's contribution to the original description in their later attribution. It may have been his lack of seniority (he was only 29 years old at the time) or his closer association with Physical Medicine than with Neurology.

Guillain described several more cases over subsequent years[17] and, in 1936,[18] set out what he considered to be the cardinal clinical features of the syndrome. The features he enumerated were as follows: 1) the sometime occurrence of a prodromal illness such as a sore throat, gastroenteritis, or malaise; 2) the neurological phase of the disease was ushered in by pain, paresthesiae, or paralysis; 3) the development of progressive flaccid paralysis, which was accentuated distally, sometimes associated with fasciculations and mild distal atrophy (it is noteworthy that, despite Guillain's characterization of the disorder as predominantly distal, it is apparent, from his own descriptions, that distal muscles were selectively involved in only four cases whereas three had predominant involvement of proximal muscles and in three the initial site of involvement was not apparent); 4) ataxia was sometimes seen; 5) tendon reflexes were lost, even in muscles that were not paralyzed; 6) there were prominent sensory symptoms but a paucity of objective changes in sensation; 7) there was occasional urinary retention or incontinence (he also noted autonomic involvement in the form of occasional disturbances in cardiac rhythm, attributing it to involvement of the tenth cranial nerve); and 8) there was cranial nerve involvement, particularly affecting the facial and extraocular nerves but also cranial nerves V, IX, X, and XII.

Guillain refused to accept as an example of this disorder any fatal case and was vehement in his rejection of any suggestion that his cases were simply nonfatal examples of Landry's paralysis. He was equally inflexible with regard to the CSF picture. He insisted that the CSF protein must be greater than 300 mg/dl and stated that it was usually much higher, although he did acknowledge that there may be "instances of an abortive form" with lower CSF protein concentration. Within 2 years of the publication of his criteria, others[19] had convincingly demonstrated that the CSF protein could be initially normal and rise to a peak as much as 35 days after the initial spinal tap. This temporal sequence was repeatedly confirmed, even during Guillain's lifetime, as reviewed by Haymaker and Kernohan.[20] Guillain also insisted that there be no increase in the CSF cell count above 10/mm³, stating, "I refuse to recognize radiculoneuritis with hyperlymphocytosis or hypernucleosis as belonging to this syndrome" (1936), another feature that has been refuted many times. CSF cell counts as high as 500/mm³ have been described[21] in otherwise typical cases and numerous reports attest to lesser degrees of pleocytosis (see Haymaker and Kernohan[20]). Thus, although the original observation of Guillain and his colleagues of albuminocytologic dissociation in the CSF was a seminal contribution to the understanding of this syndrome, his subsequent inflexibility with regard to both the clinical and CSF features of the disease tended to increase confusion rather than further the understanding of the disease.

Pathological Descriptions

The first pathological verification of the peripheral nerve as the site of pathology came in 1864, when Dumenil described the degeneration in peripheral nerves.[6] The first description of the pathological changes in peripheral nerves of patients dying of "Landry's paralysis" came about 10 years later when Dejerine and Goetz,[22] Eichorst,[23] and Van der Velden,[24] in separate accounts, described degenerative changes in the proximal parts of peripheral nerves, an anatomical location repeatedly confirmed. However, changes in the most distal nerve endings and in peripheral nerve trunks were also described, indicating the multifocal nature of the degeneration, a fact first noted in Landry's paralysis by Schmaus in 1904[25] and subsequently emphasized by Brussilowski in 1927.[26]

Early reports did not clearly distinguish between primary and secondary myelin degeneration, even though Gombault had distinguished as early as 1880 the pathological features of primary segmental demyelination from wallerian degeneration in guinea pigs chronically intoxicated with lead.[27] Even the otherwise superbly detailed pathological review of Haymaker and Kernohan in 1949 did not attempt to define the primary pathological process.[20] In 1955, Waksmann and Adams described experimental allergic neuritis (EAN) and recognized the pathological similarity of this condition to Guillain-Barré syndrome.[28] With the recognition that the primary lesion in EAN was macrophage-mediated demyelination, careful light[29] and electron[30] microscopic studies of patients who had died early during the evolution of their disease were undertaken, albeit after 14 years had elapsed. They showed pathological changes that were essentially identical to EAN.

Inflammation was recognized in the peripheral nerves from the earliest pathological descriptions,[25,31,32] but its importance in the pathogenesis of the disease went unrecognized until the 1950s. In fact, Haymaker and Kernohan[20] commented on the absence of inflammation in patients dying during the first week of illness and suggested that when present, inflammatory cells represented a reactive phenomenon. In 1969, Asbury et al.[29] found that inflammation was a quintessential feature of the disease, even in its earliest stages, and ascribed a critical pathogenetic role to lymphocytes, analogous to their role in EAN. This concept of Guillain-Barré syndrome as an autoimmune disease of a cell-mediated type remains largely unchallenged to the present (see Chapters 8 and 9).

Electrophysiological Studies

From the earliest reports of Landry[12] and of Guillain, Barré, and Strohl,[1] it was recognized that nerves and muscles retain their excitability to electrical stimuli in patients with Guillain-Barré syndrome. However, because of technical limitations, the use of electrophysiological techniques to study changes in nerve conduction in human neuropathies did not blossom until the 1950s. The finding of severe slowing of conduction velocity was first reported by Lambert in 1956,[33] and the spectrum of electrophysiological changes was reported in a large group of patients in 1964.[34] Conduction block, the quintessential feature of acute demyelination and the cause of the majority of the functional deficits in Guillain-Barré syndrome, was first implicitly inferred by Erb in 1876.[35] He found that electrical stimulation of a nerve above a focal traumatic lesion caused no visible muscular contraction whereas stimulation below the lesion produced a visible twitch. Nearly 70 years elapsed before Denny-Brown demonstrated that the pathological basis for conduction block was segmental demyelination.[36] Of course, the observations of Landry and of

Strohl, that paralyzed muscles retained the ability to contract when their nerves were electrically stimulated, we now know to be due to proximal conduction block. The first direct electrophysiological demonstration of conduction block came from the work of McDonald, who studied experimental diphtheritic lesions in the cat.[37] However, 4 years earlier, Lambert had studied several of the children reported by Peterman et al.[38] with "infectious neuronitis" and had found that "the response of a muscle was greater when the nerve was stimulated near the muscle than when it was stimulated at a distance from the muscle." In addition, he noted that there was less fibrillation than expected with needle electromyography "in harmony with other evidence that often some axons fail to conduct impulses without undergoing wallerian degeneration." It is now accepted dogma that conduction block and profound conduction slowing are the characteristic electrophysiological abnormalities in Guillain-Barré syndrome and that the former is the basis for the loss of neurological function.

Treatment

The greatest single advance in the treatment of Guillain-Barré syndrome came shortly after World War II with the development of methods of artificial ventilation. The subsequent refinement of positive pressure ventilation and the introduction of intensive care units was responsible for the dramatic fall in mortality in the 1950s. Corticosteroids were used with varying results during that same time period. However, it was the increased understanding of the disease as an autoimmune process that spurred further study of immunotherapies in the late 1970s and led to the widespread use of plasmapheresis and, more recently, high dose intravenous immunoglobulin, the first treatments to reliably influence the course of the disease.

Summary

The evolution of our appreciation of neuropathy in general and Guillain-Barré syndrome in particular has involved some of the most influential neurologists and other physicians of the 19th and 20th centuries as well as a number of obscure players. The dramatic nature of the disease has stimulated an interest out of all proportion to its prevalence. Reasonable expectations for the future include a better understanding of the immunopathogenesis of the disease and the development of more effective and safer treatments.

References

1. Guillain G, Barré A, Strohl A. Sur un syndrome de radiculonevrite avec hyperalbuminose du liquide cephalo-rachidien sans reaction cellulaire. Remarques sur les caracters cliniques et graphique des reflexes tendineux. *Bull Soc Med Hop Paris.* 1916;40:1462–1470.

2. Lettsom JC. Some remarks on the effects of Lignum Quassiae Amarae. *Mem M Soc Lond.* 1787;1:128.
3. Jackson J. On a peculiar disease resulting from the use of ardent spirits. *N Engl J Med Surg.* 1822;11:351.
4. Chomel A-F. De l'epidemie actuellement a Paris. *J Hebd Med.* 1828;1:333.
5. Graves RJ. Lecture 33: Pathology of nervous diseases. In: Neligan JM, ed. *Clinical lectures on the practice of medicine.* Dublin: Fannin and Co; 1848.
6. Dumenil L. Paralysie peripherique du mouvement et du sentiment portant sur les quartres membres. Atrophie des rameaux nerveux des parties paralysees. *Gaz Hebd Med.* 1864; 1:203–207.
7. Dumenil L. Contributions pour servir a l'histoire des paralysies peripheriques, et specialement de la nevrite. *Gaz Hebd Med.* 1866;3:51–84.
8. Vulpian E-F-A. *Maladies du systeme nerveux: maladies de la moelle.* Paris: O Doin; 1879.
9. Viets HR. History of peripheral neuritis as a clinical entity. *Arch Neurol Psychiatry.* 1934; 32:377–394.
10. Wardrop J. Clinical observations on various diseases. *Lancet.* 1834;1:380.
11. Ollivier C-P. *Traite des maladies de la moelle epiniere.* Vol. 2., 3rd ed. Paris: Mequignon-Marvis Pere et Fils; 1837.
12. Landry O. Note sur la paralysie ascendante aigue. *Gaz Hebd Med.* 1859;6:472–474, 486–488.
13. Fisher M. An unusual variant of acute idiopathic polyneuritis (syndrome of ophthalmoplegia, ataxia and areflexia). *N Engl J Med.* 1956;255:57–65.
14. Roemheld L. Zur klinik postdiphtherischer pseudotabes; liquorbefunde bei postdiphtherischer lahmung. *Dtsch Med Wochenschr.* 1908;35:669–671.
15. Queckenstedt HG. Uber veranderungen der spinalflussigkeit bei erkrankunger peripherer nerven, insbesondere bei polyneuritis und bei ischias. *Dtsch Ztschr Nervenh.* 1917;57:316–329.
16. Draganescu S, Claudian J. Sur un cas de radiculo-nevrite curable (syndrome de Guillain-Barré) apparue au cours d'une osteo-myelite du bras. *Rev Neurol.* 1927;2:517–521.
17. Guillain G, Alajouanine T, Perisson J. Sur le syndrome de radiculo-nevrite aigue curable avec dissociation albuminocytologique du liquide cephalo-radichien. *Rev Neurol.* 1925;1:492–507.
18. Guillain G. Radiculoneuritis with acellular hyperalbuminosis of the cerebrospinal fluid. *Arch Neurol Psychiatry.* 1936;36:975–990.
19. Madigan PS, Marietta SU. Polyradiculoneuritis, with report of a case. *Ann Intern Med.* 1938;12:719.
20. Haymaker W, Kernohan JW. The Landry-Guillain-Barré syndrome. A clinicopathologic report of fifty fatal cases and a critique of the literature. *Medicine.* 1949;28:59–141.
21. Mussio-Fournier JC, Cervino JM, Rocca F, Larossa-Helguera RA. Un cas de meningoradiculo-nevrite aigue curable, avec xanthochromie et intense lymphocytose dans liquide cephalo-radichien, se terminant par une guerison complete. *Rev Neurol.* 1933;2:104.
22. Dejerine J, Goetz A. Note sur un cas de paralysie ascendante aigue. *Arch Physiol.* 1876;8:312–322.
23. Eichorst H. Neuritis acuta progressiva. *Virch Arch Pathol Anat.* 1877;69:265–274.
24. Van der Velden R. Ein fall von acuter aufsteigender spinaler paralyse. *Dtsch Arch Klin Med.* 1877;19:333.
25. Schmaus H. Die Landryschen paralyse. *Ergebn Allg Path Path Anat.* 1904;9:396–422.
26. Brussilowski L. Zur lehre von der akuten aufsteigenden Landryschen paralyse. *Zentralblatt Ges Neurol Psychiatrie.* 1927;111:515–528.
27. Gombault A. Contribution a l'etude anatomique de la nevrite parenchymateuse subaigue et chronique—nevrite segmentaire peri-axile. *Arch Neurol (Paris).* 1880;1:11.
28. Waksman BH, Adams RA. Allergic neuritis: an experimental disease of rabbits induced by the injection of peripheral nervous tissue and adjuvants. *J Exp Med.* 1955;102:213–235.
29. Asbury AK, Arnason BG, Adams RD. The inflammatory lesion in idiopathic polyneuritis. Its role in pathogenesis. *Medicine.* 1969;48:173–215.
30. Wisniewski H, Terry RD, Whitaker JN, Cook SD, Dowling PC. Landry-Guillain-Barré syndrome. A primary demyelinating disease. *Arch Neurol.* 1969;21:269–276.
31. Hoffmann J. Ein fall von acuter aufsteigender paralyse. *Arch Psychiatry.* 1884;15:140.
32. Thomas JJ. Two cases of acute ascending paralysis, with autopsy. *Am J Med Sci.* 1898;116:133–148.
33. Lambert EH. Electromyography and electrical stimulation of peripheral nerve and muscle. In: *Mayo Clinic and Mayo Foundation. Clinical examinations in neurology.* Philadelphia: Saunders; 1956.

34. Lambert EH, Mulder DW. Nerve conduction in the Guillain-Barré syndrome. *Electroenceph Clin Neurophysiol*. 1964;17:86.
35. Erb WF. Diseases of the cerebrospinal nerves. In: von Ziemssen H, ed. *Cyclopaedia of the practice of medicine*. London: Sampson, Lowe, Marston, Searle and Rivington; 1876.
36. Denny-Brown D, Brenner C. Paralysis of nerve induced by direct pressure and by tourniquet. *Arch Neurol Psychiatry*. 1944;51:1–26.
37. McDonald WI. The effects of experimental demyelination on conduction of peripheral nerve: a histological and electrophysiological study: II. Electrophysiological observations. *Brain*. 1963;86:501–524.
38. Peterman AF, Daly DD, Dion FR, Keith HM. Infectious neuronitis (Guillain-Barré syndrome) in children. *Neurology*. 1959;9:533–539.

2

Clinical Features of Guillain-Barré Syndrome

Guillain-Barré syndrome (GBS) has become the most common cause of acute paralysis in Western countries since the virtual elimination of poliomyelitis with vaccination programs. Nonetheless it remains a rare disease and, although its classical clinical features are well recognized, diagnosis is often delayed by a failure to recognize the less typical clinical presentations. The development of treatments, which are most effective when started within a week of onset of symptoms, has made early diagnosis imperative and a thorough knowledge of the diverse presentations of this syndrome important.

Typical Clinical Features

Motor Abnormalities

GBS is a predominantly motor neuropathy (Tables 2–1 and 2–2), a feature noted repeatedly from its earliest descriptions,[1-9] and may appear to be purely motor by clinical criteria. Weakness usually begins in the legs. It is nearly always bilateral and most reports emphasize its relative symmetry. However, in our experience, some degree of asymmetry is common and it is occasionally striking. At the time of presentation, the paralysis is usually distally accentuated and involves the legs before the arms ("ascending paralysis"), but the spread is not strictly contiguous, a fact noted by Landry[1] in his original description. Although most reports have emphasized this distal

Table 2–1. Frequency of Motor Abnormalities in GBS*

	% OF PATIENTS
Limb weakness	98
Proximal more	15
Distal more	35
Both equal	50
Cranial weakness	
III, IV, VI	8
V	10
VII	49
X	16
XI	8
XII	5
Respiratory insufficiency	
Reduced vital capacity only	8
Required ventilation	23

*In more than 600 patients from six series published over the last three decades.[4,6,7,9,10,17]

accentuation, Ropper and Shahani found proximal leg weakness to be actually more frequent and more prominent than distal.[10] The hands and arms usually become involved, although somewhat later in the course of progression. At the nadir of the illness there is approximately equal weakness of proximal and distal muscles in about half of the cases. The paralyzed limbs are flaccid, in proportion to the weakness. Fasciculations are occasionally seen. Facial and limb myokymia is not uncommon. Mateer et al.[11] noted clinical myokymia, confirmed by needle electromyography (EMG), in 17% of unselected cases of GBS, all but one involving the facial muscles. Others have also noted the presence of myokymia.[12–15] Painful muscular rigidity with abnormal "pseudospastic" posturing has also been described, associated with peripherally generated, continuous motor unit activity recorded by needle EMG.[16] Muscle atrophy would not be expected early in the course of the disease, although Winer et al. noted it in 56% of patients at the time of presentation.[17] Later it is frequent, at least in severe cases, both because of disuse atrophy, occurring in paralyzed muscles, and because axonal degeneration commonly accompanies the demyelination.

Table 2–2. Unusual Motor Abnormalities

Fasciculations
Myokymia
Pseudospasticity
Ptosis

In severe cases (about 30%), abdominal and thoracic muscles, including the diaphragm, are involved leading to compromised respiratory reserve and eventual respiratory failure. Weakness of the respiratory muscles leads to a reduction in both vital capacity and tidal volume. In addition, there is reduced sighing, which is an important cause of atelectasis. This problem is compounded by poor coughing and sometimes by the associated bulbar weakness, which may result in aspiration. The atelectasis produces shunting of blood between arterial and venous circulations resulting in mild hypoxemia. The resultant tachypnea actually reduces the pco_2 in the same way that pulmonary embolism does. Thus, the earliest sign of impending respiratory failure is the development of mild hypoxia and hypocapnea, not hypercapnea. Nonetheless, hypoventilation and hypercapnea eventually supervene if the earlier signs of respiratory failure are not recognized. The increased muscular effort associated with tachypnea leads to further fatigue of respiratory muscles and accelerates the progression of respiratory failure.

Cranial innervated muscles are often involved leading to dysphagia, dysarthria, facial diplegia, and diplopia. Facial diplegia can be found in more than 50% of cases if it is carefully sought. Laryngeal and pharyngeal weakness is fortunately uncommon but has important implications for prognosis and management. Minor dysphagia may lead to aspiration if it is not recognized and laryngeal weakness contributes to poor coughing and difficulty with clearing secretions. Extraocular involvement is less common (<10%); the abducens nerve is the most commonly involved. Ptosis and pupillary abnormalities are rarely seen. Occasionally, in the most severe cases, there is almost complete paralysis of peripheral, axial, respiratory, and cranial muscles and a "locked-in" state may result with the patient fully alert and orientated and yet unable to communicate except, on some occasions, with eye movements.[18,19]

Weakness usually progresses over 1 to 3 weeks, although the nadir is often reached earlier, particularly in mild cases. The National Institute of Neurological and Communicative Disorders and Stroke (NINCDS) diagnostic criteria exclude cases in which progression exceeds 3 weeks. Nonetheless, progression over longer periods occasionally occurs in otherwise typical cases but should raise questions about the diagnosis. Once the nadir is reached there is a variable interval before recovery begins, with improvement occurring earlier and more rapidly in mild cases. The rate and degree of recovery of function depend primarily on the amount of associated axonal degeneration. Patients with mild weakness, normal amplitude of distally elicited compound muscle action potentials on nerve conduction studies, and few fibrillation potentials with needle EMG have almost pure demyelination and recover rapidly and completely, within about 12 to 20 weeks. Even with severe weakness, if motor amplitudes are normal and there are few fibrillations, complete recovery usually occurs, although its time course may be somewhat longer. When there is evidence of severe axonal degeneration with low amplitude or unelicitable motor responses on nerve conduction studies and profuse fibrillation with needle EMG, time for recovery is protracted, sometimes taking as much as 2 years, and recovery is usually incomplete. However, even these severely involved patients usually recover sufficient function to walk independently.[20]

Sensory Abnormalities

Although weakness is the most prominent feature of GBS, in about 60% to 70% of cases the onset of the disease is heralded by the development of distal paresthesiae and sometimes pain and muscle cramping (see Table 2–3). This early pain usually has a deep aching quality and may be severe. Painful paresthesiae may also occur but usually appear later. Lancinating and burning pains are infrequent. Pain is a greatly underappreciated symptom in GBS and yet it has been frequently cited. It was the presenting symptom in one of the original cases reported by Guillain and his colleagues[2] and has been described as affecting up to 83% of cases, although a lower frequency (30–50%) has usually been reported.[7,21–23] It is typically poorly localized but is accentuated proximally, in the back, posterior thighs, and shoulder girdle, although almost any anatomical site may be affected. There may be muscle cramps and muscles are often tender to palpation. The pathogenesis of the pain is obscure but it has been suggested that it may be due to activation of nociceptive afferents arising from the nerve trunks themselves (nervi nervorum), perhaps as the result of inflammation and edema.[24] Alternatively, the pain may be related to myonecrosis, since the serum creatine kinase is often elevated in patients with severe pain,[20] or to spontaneous firing of demyelinated axons.[25]

Although paresthesiae are common, objective sensory loss is usually trivial, even when paralysis is severe. However, objective sensory loss does occur and occasionally is a prominent feature.[8,9] Ravn[8] suggested that sensory loss was more common than was generally appreciated but that, because

Table 2–3. Frequency of Sensory Abnormalities*

	% OF PATIENTS
Sensory symptoms	
Numbness/paresthesiae	72
Pain	37
Sensory signs	62
Reflexes	
Normal	5
Partial loss	17
Complete loss	78

*In more than 600 patients from six series published over the last three decades.[4,6,7,9,10,17]

it was overshadowed by paralysis, was underreported. This view is supported by reports from series of patients who were carefully examined in whom objective sensory loss was found in 60% to 85% of patients.[6,7] The infrequency of objective sensory loss reported in children (<30%) may also reflect difficulty with the examination.[6] Sensory modalities mediated by the large myelinated axons are usually the most prominently involved.[5] Vibration sensation and proprioception may be lost or reduced in the distal extremities, sometimes to a severe degree. Severe loss of proprioception may lead to a sensory ataxia and pseudoathetosis. This may be attributed to cerebellar involvement leading to the incorrect assumption of central nervous system (CNS) involvement or even an incorrect diagnosis. Proprioceptive loss is almost certainly the cause of ataxia in the Fisher variant of GBS, as will be discussed later.

Areflexia or hyporeflexia is almost invariable in GBS, reflecting involvement of large diameter muscle spindle afferent axons, usually in the dorsal root. It is usually seen at the time of presentation, even when other signs are trivial, and occurs even in areas apparently otherwise unaffected. Although the reflexes may be normal early in the course of the paralysis, the persistence of completely normal reflexes is rare, occurring in less than 5% of patients. In a patient suspected of having GBS, preservation of reflexes should give pause and other diagnostic possibilities should be seriously considered. For example, we have seen several patients with acutely evolving paralysis from an acute motor neuron syndrome, referred for evaluation of GBS. In each, a clue to the correct diagnosis was the persistent preservation of reflexes.

The sensations of pain, temperature, and light touch are usually relatively preserved although a subjective alteration in the quality of cutaneous stimulation is often noted. Severe loss of cutaneous sensibility, particularly when strength is relatively preserved, should raise significant questions about the diagnosis. Occasionally a graded sensory loss may extend up onto the lower trunk but the presence of a definite sensory level is inconsistent with a diagnosis of GBS.

A pure sensory variant of GBS has been described. The most convincing case was reported by Dawson et al.,[26] who were afforded the opportunity to perform an autopsy study. Their patient had severe, acute sensory loss, particularly affecting proprioception, with only mild weakness. The spinal fluid showed typical albuminocytologic dissociation. At autopsy there was severe inflammatory demyelination, concentrated in the dorsal roots, but also affecting peripheral nerves. Ventral roots were spared and sections taken from multiple sites in the brain and spinal cord were normal. Although clinically atypical, this case showed the quintessential pathological features of GBS, namely inflammatory demyelination of peripheral nerves, unusual only in its distribution. However, for most of the other reported cases with predominantly sensory features, the evidence is poor that immune-mediated demyelination is the basis for symptoms and signs. The syndrome of acute or subacute sensory loss is most often caused by an acute sensory ganglioneuropathy, a disorder described in Chapter 3, which superficially resembles GBS. This disorder is characterized by acute inflammation and neuronal degeneration involving the dorsal root ganglion, rather than by macrophage-mediated demyelination of peripheral nerves.

Autonomic Abnormalities

Autonomic neuropathy (Table 2–4) in GBS, like pain, is underappreciated by most neurologists, although it has been long recognized. Several large published series of cases have completely ignored the autonomic features or have relegated them to a few casual comments.[6,9,27] Much of the residual mortality of GBS that has persisted since the introduction of effective ventilatory support is attributable to autonomic instability. Death in Landry's patient reported in 1869 may have been due to arrhythmia exacerbated by hypoxia since it was sudden and did not appear to be due to respiratory failure alone.[2] Osler specifically referred to "paralysis of the heart" as a cause of death in acute febrile polyneuritis.[28] Some form of autonomic disturbance has been reported in 100% of cases with specific and sensitive testing, although fortunately it is usually not life-threatening.[29] In some series, autonomic instability was found only in those patients requiring artificial ventilation.[30] However, others have reported that it is not confined to patients with respiratory failure or severe paralysis, although it is usually more prominent in patients with more severe disease.[29,31,32] Because of the risk of sudden death from serious but treatable cardiac arrhythmias, it is important to monitor closely whenever possible all but the mildest cases of GBS.

The changes may be clinically trivial, such as altered acral sweating (both increased and decreased) and changes in vasomotor control leading to acral cyanosis, both of which occur frequently. For example, Appenzeller and Marshall found seven of eight patients had abnormal vasomotor control even though none had symptoms.[33] Similarly, constipation and urinary hesitancy are common, proceeding to urinary retention in some cases and occasionally

Table 2–4. Frequency of Autonomic Instability*

	% OF PATIENTS
Urinary dysfunction	25
Rectal dysfunction	14
Hypotension	14
Hypertension	31
Sinus tachycardia (> 90/min)	36
Arrhythmia	16
Hyponatremia (SIADH)	9

*Estimated from two large series[30,32] and other reports of smaller numbers of patients.[29,31,44]

to paralytic ileus. Less frequently there is severe and potentially life-threatening autonomic instability. Postural hypotension is common and may lead to loss of consciousness on occasions. Birchfield and Shaw[34] described postural hypotension in three of six patients, two of whom presented with syncope and had severe postural blood pressure changes documented. Lichtenfeld[31] found some evidence suggestive of insufficient sympathetic activity in 100% of 28 patients, 12 of whom were evaluated prospectively and the remainder from a review of their charts. Twelve patients had documented postural hypotension, which usually occurred early in the illness, and in two it was the presenting symptom. Four of these patients failed to develop a compensatory tachycardia when their blood pressure fell. The remainder had lesser degrees of sympathetic insufficiency but in many it consisted of symptoms gleaned from a review of patient records, without objective confirmation. Hypertension, which may be sustained but which is more often paroxysmal and alternates with marked hypotension, also occurs and may be severe enough to require treatment. Lichtenfeld found hypertension in 17 of 28 patients that lasted from 2 to 21 days and went up as high as 260/160. He found no correlation between elevated blood pressure and elevated levels of circulating catecholamines, but Davies and Dingle[35] found increased catecholamines in four of five patients with hypertension with reversion to normal as the hypertension improved, and others have corroborated these findings.[36,37] More recently, it has been suggested that the elevated blood pressure might be due to increased release of atrial natriuretic factor in response to high circulating catecholamines.[38,39] Laufer et al.[40] describe a case of GBS with hypertension without other signs of sympathetic overactivity in whom there was marked elevation of plasma renin. Treatment with propanolol reduced plasma renin activity to normal and abolished the hypertension. Because the blood pressure may vacillate widely between hypertension and hypotension, extreme care must be exercised in treating blood pressure changes and nonpharmacological treatment or treatment with intravenous drugs with a short duration of action is preferable.

A variety of abnormalities of cardiac rhythm may also occur in association with GBS. It should be emphasized that not all of these are due to autonomic neuropathy but may be due to hypoxia, pulmonary embolism, or infection. In addition, arrhythmias may occur as a result of focal myocarditis, which has been reported in patients with GBS.[21,41] However, arrhythmias may also occur as the sole manifestation of autonomic instability. Abnormal heart rate variation with respiration or the Valsalva maneuver, even in the absence of overt arrhythmia, can be demonstrated in practically all patients with GBS.[29,42,43] Greenland and Griggs[44] reported overt abnormalities of cardiac rhythm in 13 of 16 consecutive monitored patients admitted to an intensive care unit with GBS. These included atrioventricular (AV) block (eight patients), sinus tachycardia (eight), sinus bradycardia (five), sinus arrest (two), atrial flutter or fibrillation (six), and even brief episodes of ventricular tachycardia (four). Most were asymptomatic but two patients with AV block and sinus arrest required treatment with a demand pacemaker. These patients may not be representative of all GBS patients since they all had disease severe enough to necessitate admission to the intensive care unit but they do underscore the importance of close observation of GBS patients. A number of other case reports attest to the occurrence of bradyarrhythmias, sometimes necessitating cardiac demand pacing.[45-48] Other signs of abnormal parasympathetic activity may also occur in association with these bradyarrhythmias, manifested as flushing, tightness in the chest, and increased production of bronchial secretions. In older patients this may be mistaken for myocardial ischemia or cardiac failure. This confusion may be compounded by the dramatic abnormalities of the electrocardiograph, which occasionally occur in GBS without other evidence of myocardial damage.[31,44,49] Persistent sinus tachycardia is very common, occurring in all of the patients evaluated by Tuck and McLeod[29] and in half of those reported by Lichtenfeld.[31] Paroxysmal sinus tachycardia may also occur, sometimes associated with diaphoresis and peripheral vasoconstriction. More serious cardiac arrhythmias such as atrial tachycardia, atrial fibrillation, and ventricular tachycardia are less common. Succinylcholine, often used to produce muscle relaxation to facilitate endotracheal intubation, should be avoided in patients with GBS since it may precipitate dangerous arrhythmias.[50] Even mild but sustained hypoxia in GBS patients may exacerbate cardiac arrhythmias. Therefore, early intervention should be considered in patients with limited respiratory reserve, to diminish the risk of these hypoxia-related arrhythmias.

Another rare complication of GBS that may be related to the autonomic neuropathy is inappropriate secretion of antidiuretic hormone (ADH) resulting in hyponatremia. Severe hyponatremia with encephalopathy and seizures, complicating typical GBS, was first described in four patients by Posner et al. in 1967.[51] All patients met the clinical criteria for inappropriate ADH secretion as the cause of their hyponatremia: they had increased specific gravity of urine and increased sodium excretion in the face of hyponatremia. It was suggested that the inappropriate ADH secretion resulted from neuropathic involvement of the autonomic afferent fibers arising from vascular stretch receptors. Penney et al.[52] evaluated a patient with hyponatremia associated with GBS and found that responses to a water load and to infusion of hypertonic saline were essentially normal. They suggested that the hyponatremia in their patient resulted from a resetting of osmoreceptors. Transient diabetes insipidus has also been described in GBS. Polydipsia and polyuria resolved concomitant with resolution of the neuropathy.[53]

With the tremendous improvement in care of ventilator dependent patients over the last one to two decades, autonomic instability has become a major contributor to morbidity and mortality in GBS. It is also important to recognize the potential for the occurrence of autonomic instability during plasmapheresis, which has become almost universally used for treatment of GBS and which may exacerbate labile blood pressure and the tendency toward arrhythmias.

Although autonomic neuropathy is a frequent finding in GBS, it is equally important to recognize that complications such as pulmonary embolism and infections, especially pneumonia, may produce cardiac arrhythmias and changes in blood pressure that may mimic autonomic instability. In addition, the earliest signs of respiratory failure are very similar. It is obviously critical to be able to distinguish these complications from autonomic neuropathy so that appropriate early treatment can be instituted.

Atypical and Restricted Forms of GBS

Miller-Fisher Syndrome

In 1956, Fisher described a syndrome of ataxia, areflexia, and ophthalmoplegia and suggested that it was a variant of GBS.[54] In all three of his cases there was severe external and mild internal ophthalmoplegia and profound ataxia beginning about a week after an antecedent infectious illness. Although the ophthalmoplegia and ataxia dominated the clinical picture, all patients became areflexic, one had a profound loss of vibratory perception, mild cutaneous insensibility, and weakness, and one had prominent paresthesiae. The cerebrospinal fluid was examined in two of the patients on more than one occasion in each. In one it was normal initially and then rose sharply, whereas in the other it was normal throughout the illness. All patients spontaneously recovered. Although this report is often cited as the original description of this variant, previous authors had described the same clinical features earlier.[55,56] Numerous subsequent reports have confirmed the essential features of the syndrome as detailed by Fisher, in adults[57–59] and in children.[60,61] The degree of involvement of other cranial nerves and peripheral motor, sensory, and autonomic functions has varied but dominance of the original triad has been used to define this unusual variant of GBS. Many patients who present with this initial restricted cranial nerve involvement progress to develop more generalized GBS and many patients with severe GBS develop the essential features of this variant as a part of their clinical picture during the evolution of their disease. The potential for deterioration necessitating assisted ventilation and the occasional occurrence of autonomic instability are important to recognize in a syndrome that is often considered to be a relatively benign variant of GBS.[62,63]

The pathogenesis of the ataxia in Miller-Fisher syndrome has generated considerable controversy. Many believe this ataxia has a cerebellar basis and consider it a part of a brain stem encephalitis that can manifest itself with signs of supranuclear extraocular paralysis, abnormalities of brain stem auditory evoked potentials, alterations in level of consciousness, and other abnormalities of mental status. Al-Din et al.[64] describe a group of 18 patients which appears to be far from homogeneous. All had ophthalmoplegia and ataxia but only 11 developed areflexia. The other six had increased reflexes and extensor plantar responses and are unlikely to have been mistaken for GBS, in any form. Even many of the 11 areflexic patients were atypical for GBS. Three had significant CSF pleocytosis and three others had significant alteration of the level of consciousness, one of whom had seizures. Like the Miller-Fisher syndrome, the prognosis was excellent. Although most of these patients probably did not have GBS, this report emphasizes that not all patients with the classical triad of ophthalmoplegia, ataxia, and areflexia have a primarily neuropathic disorder. Others have emphasized the frequency with which the ophthalmoplegia had the characteristics of a supranuclear palsy in suggesting a central origin for the findings.[65,66] Further support for a possible central origin of the ataxia and ophthalmoplegia comes from the occasional abnormalities reported with computerized tomography[64,67,68] and abnormalities involving central conduction pathways of the brain stem auditory evoked potential.[69] Others have argued strongly that the ataxia can be more easily explained on the basis of abnormal proprioceptive function and that it is unnecessary to invoke abnormalities of the CNS.[70–72] Ropper argues persuasively that apparent supranuclear eye movement disorders may be seen in peripheral disorders that are unequivocally confined to the peripheral (neuromuscular) system, such as myasthenia gravis. Many multimodality evoked potential studies on patients with Miller-Fisher syndrome have failed to demonstrate evidence of disruption of central pathways of auditory or somatic sensation.[70,73] Landau et al.[74] and Ropper[75] obtained magnetic resonance imaging at the height of the illness in several patients and again found no abnormalities, arguing strongly against a cerebellar lesion or brain stem lesions as the cause of the clinical syndrome. Finally, clinicopathological studies have been carried out on two patients with Miller-Fisher syndrome and in both the only abnormality was inflammatory demyelination of peripheral occulomotor nerves with no CNS pathology.[76,77] Thus, it is clear that it is not necessary to invoke involvement of the CNS to explain the ataxia or other clinical features in Miller-Fisher syndrome. However, there may be a syndrome of brain stem encephalitis in which there is peripheral nerve involvement. Perhaps a viral syndrome in which one of the features is brain stem encephalitis may trigger, in some patients, a postinfectious neuropathy.

There is also some controversy concerning the nature of the neuropathy in Miller-Fisher syndrome. Most reports have supported the initial contention that this is a primary demyelinating neuropathy with cranial nerve involvement. This conclusion has been based on the occasional observations of slow conduction velocity, sometimes with conduction block, electrodiagnostic features characteristic of demyelination. However, Fross and Daube[78] reviewed the electrodiagnostic features of 10 patients from the Mayo Clinic as well as those contained within six reports from the literature. The patients had classical clinical features of Miller-Fisher syndrome. They found the electrodiagnostic features to be more characteristic of an axonal neuropathy; namely, low amplitude sensory and motor evoked responses, with little slowing, and evidence of mild denervation on the EMG. Furthermore, changes were more prominent in sensory nerves. They felt that the pattern of abnormalities was distinct from that seen in typical GBS and concluded that they were the result of an axonal neuropathy or sensory neuropathy. However, the rapidity and efficacy of recovery from the neurological deficits and the profound, often global, areflexia argue strongly in favor of a major demyelinating component to the pathology in most patients with this syndrome. A syndrome of recurrent sensory neuropathy and ophthalmoplegia, perhaps akin to Miller-Fisher syndrome, has also been described.[79,80]

GBS with Proximally Accentuated Weakness

Although classically described as an ascending paralysis, GBS frequently presents with weakness that equally affects proximal and distal muscles or is even proximally accentuated. As far back as 1865, Pellegrino-Levy[81] noted the sometime occurrence of descending paralysis. More recently, in the series reported by Ropper and Shahani,[10] only about half of the patients had more lower than upper extremity weakness. In about 30% of patients there was equal involvement of upper and lower limbs and in 12% the arms were more affected. Furthermore, within a limb, weakness may be more severe in proximal than distal muscles and axial and respiratory muscles may be involved when distal weakness is trivial. Occasionally respiratory compromise may be the initial manifestation of the weakness.

Cranial nerves are frequently involved in advanced cases but may also be involved when distal weakness is absent or minimal. In rare instances paralysis begins in cranial innervated muscles causing ophthalmoplegia, facial diplegia or bulbar palsy before limb weakness. Such cases may be mistaken for botulism, myasthenia gravis, rabies, or diphtheria. Facial paralysis is the most common cranial nerve manifestation, occurring at some stage in the evolution of the disease in more than 50% of cases, and it is not necessarily confined to cases with severe limb weakness. It is usually bilateral but may be strikingly asymmetrical. Other cranial nerves are also often involved, sometimes without much peripheral weakness. As already mentioned, in the Miller-Fisher syndrome there is primary involvement of the oculomotor nerves, all of which may also be involved in other clinical forms either together or individually. Trigeminal involvement is rare but facial numbness or paresthesiae and difficulty chewing may occur. Deafness has also been reported rarely. In one case there was complete loss of all waves of the brain stem auditory evoked response, which returned with markedly prolonged latency, coincident with the return of hearing.[82] The lower cranial nerves may also be involved causing dysphagia, dysarthria, and difficulty lifting the head. Even when there is accentuation of proximal weakness in GBS, sensory symptoms and signs still tend to be accentuated distally.

With this occasional accentuation of proximal weakness it is important to recognize that respiratory or bulbar paralysis may be the initial manifestation of the neuropathy or can occur when distal weakness is still quite mild.

Therefore, all patients must be monitored closely for signs of respiratory failure or bulbar dysfunction regardless of the apparent severity of the disease as judged by the degree of distal weakness.

GBS with Asymmetric Weakness

Symmetrical involvement from side to side is usually reported in patients with GBS but, since the syndrome is characterized by multifocal pathology, it is not surprising that clinical evidence of that multifocality is often apparent. Mild asymmetry is almost always encountered if it is specifically sought and strikingly asymmetric cases occur. At least at the outset, a monomelic or hemiplegic distribution of weakness may be seen. In almost all cases bilateral involvement appears as the disease progresses. However, in the interests of early diagnosis and treatment, recognition of the initial focal manifestations is important.

GBS with Prominent Axonal Degeneration

There have been several recent reports of a syndrome clinically indistinguishable from GBS but in which the electrodiagnostic features and pathological studies indicate that the primary abnormality is axonal degeneration rather than demyelination, as is usually seen in GBS.[83–85] The cases fulfilled enough of the NINCDS criteria for the diagnosis of GBS; namely, acutely evolving paralysis with trivial or absent sensory abnormalities, areflexia or hyporeflexia, and elevated CSF protein (in most cases). They could be distinguished electrophysiologically from typical GBS because of inexcitable motor nerves or very low amplitude motor responses during the acute phase of the illness, and the development of profound spontaneous activity, indicating severe axonal degeneration, as the disease progressed. This entity has a poor prognosis with all of the described patients dying or remaining severely disabled, many respirator dependent. At autopsy, there was severe, widespread axonal degeneration with little demyelination and no inflammation. Whether this acute paralytic illness should be considered a variant of GBS on pathogenetic grounds is controversial since the pathologic *sine qua non* of GBS is macrophage-mediated demyelination. However, the clinical similarity is striking and it is important to recognize that not all cases of acute paralysis have as good a prognosis as typical GBS.

Central Nervous System Involvement in GBS

Although there is a universal consensus that GBS is primarily a disease of the peripheral nervous system, there is controversy concerning both the frequency and the significance of CNS involvement. There is no doubt that there may be clinical or laboratory evidence of CNS involvement in GBS (see Table

Table 2–5.   Suggested CNS Manifestations of GBS

Papilledema (5%)
Optic neuritis
Encephalopathy (obtundation, confusion, seizures)
Myelopathy
Aseptic meningitis
Supranuclear eye movement disorders
Ataxia
SIADH

2–5), but the pathogenesis of the various abnormalities is unknown. It is unlikely that these abnormalities result from an immune-mediated attack on CNS myelin.

GBS with Papilledema (Pseudotumor Cerebri)

Papilledema is a well described but uncommon accompaniment of GBS, occurring in up to 5% of patients, particularly in children.[86] It is most commonly seen in patients with severe elevation of CSF protein, leading Denny-Brown[87] and others[88] to suggest that the high CSF protein concentration might inhibit resorption of CSF by the arachnoid villi. However, it has been reported even with only mild CSF protein elevation. In a study of 31 patients with acute, chronic, or relapsing demyelinating neuropathies with papilledema, Morley and Reynolds[89] found that the CSF protein was elevated above 400 mg/dl in only half and in four patients it was less than 200 mg/dl. In addition, the coincidental onset of papilledema and the neuropathy has been described with normal initial CSF protein, which rose only later in the course of the disease.[90] Furthermore, even when the lumbar spinal fluid protein concentration is profoundly elevated, the cisternal concentration is much less and, presumably, the concentration over the convexity, where CSF absorption is taking place, is even less. Therefore, the concept that the high CSF protein concentration is somehow restricting CSF absorption into the blood stream through arachnoid granulations cannot explain the occurrence of the raised intracranial pressure in GBS, and the CSF protein per se is unlikely to be the primary determinant of papilledema. The situation is analogous to pseudotumor cerebri, and studies of CSF dynamics in patients with GBS have shown normal production rates with reduced outflow as is found in other patients with pseudotumor cerebri.[91–93] However, the increased resistance to outflow seems insufficient to account totally for the magnitude of the intracranial hypertension and other factors may also play an important role. For example, Joynt[94] reported the presence of cerebral edema without inflammation or demyelination in the brain biopsy of a child with GBS and papilledema.

GBS with Optic Neuritis

There have been several case reports of GBS associated with optic neuritis, either as an isolated CNS abnormality or associated with other CNS findings.[95–100] In two instances, optic neuritis alone or optic neuritis associated with transverse myelitis occurred 4 weeks before the onset of typical GBS.[100] This temporal relationship led to the suggestion that the optic neuritis resulted in release of myelin antigens common to both CNS and peripheral nervous system (PNS) and produced a secondary, immune-mediated demyelination of peripheral nerve. However, the infrequency of the association suggests that it may be no more than coincidental.

Encephalopathy in GBS

The most commonly reported CNS abnormality in GBS is alteration in mental status, often associated with abnormalities of the electroencephalogram, suggesting an encephalopathy. Obtundation and confusion may be accompanied by seizures. However, these abnormalities are more likely to have an alternative explanation in most cases. Hypoxia and hypercapnea in patients with overt or incipient respiratory failure, sometimes associated with the use of a sedative or other drugs, is a common cause. The syndrome of inappropriate secretion of ADH with hyponatremia may also account for some cases of altered mental status and seizures. Some patients in whom the encephalopathy occurs in close temporal proximity to the onset of the paralysis may have a persistent encephalitis related to an antecedent viral infection. In others, with severe disease, a psychological reaction to the paralysis or confinement to the intensive care unit may result in confusion or other signs that may be mistaken for encephalopathy.

Features of encephalopathy, with obtundation and seizures, may be more common in children and has led some to designate the syndrome as an encephalomyeloradiculoneuropathy, a term as clumsy as it is inaccurate for most cases.[101,102] Encephalopathy in children with GBS typically occurs early in the course of the illness,[103,104] which suggests that it may be part of the prodromal viral illness with encephalitis, rather than a CNS participation in the subsequent immunological response. Acute, severe, combined, demyelination (ASCD) of the central and peripheral nervous systems has been suggested as a distinct clinical entity occurring in children. There have been two cases reported in children of the simultaneous onset of acute disseminated encephalomyelitis and GBS.[105,106] The former was established by a characteristic picture with magnetic resonance imaging (MRI) and the latter with nerve conduction studies. Both patients recovered completely and rapidly coincident with corticosteroid treatment. Similar cases have been described in adults,[107,108] in which the autopsy revealed acute, macrophage-mediated demyelination of both the CNS and PNS. It has been suggested that these cases constitute a simultaneous attack on central and peripheral myelin as a result of cross-antigenicity.

Myelopathy in GBS

Extensor plantar responses are occasionally found in patients with GBS and, rarely, patients may have a sensory level on the trunk. However, truncal sensory loss is usually a graded one, rather than a distinct sensory level, and is more likely to arise from peripheral nerve involvement. There is no incontrovertible clinical evidence of spinal cord involvement in patients with GBS, although small collections of perivascular lymphocytes are occasionally found in the spinal cord of fatal cases.[21]

Aseptic Meningitis

Some early authors were sufficiently impressed by the clinical signs of meningeal irritation to designate the syndrome as a meningoradiculoneuritis. However, many of these earlier cases were poorly characterized and may have been atypical cases of poliomyelitis or some other infectious process. A few lymphocytes in the CSF are often seen in otherwise typical cases and occasionally there is a marked pleocytosis, especially early in the course of the disease. In patients dying of GBS some meningeal inflammation has also been seen. However, in the great majority of cases there is neither clinical nor pathological evidence of significant meningeal involvement.

Supranuclear Eye Movement Disorders and Ataxia

As previously discussed, several authors have noted an apparent supranuclear eye movement disorder in patients with GBS. For example, Bell's phenomenon of preserved upward rotation of the eyes with attempted eye closure may be seen in patients who lack volitional upward gaze. Other patients have had preserved convergence, in the face of paralysis of adduction, and even features of an internuclear ophthalmoplegia have been described.[65] However, this entire range of eye movement disorders may also occasionally be seen in myasthenia gravis so, without excluding the possibility of CNS pathology, it is clearly not essential to invoke central lesions to explain these abnormalities. Ataxia has also been invoked as evidence of CNS involvement but is more likely to be a sensory ataxia due to involvement of proprioceptive afferents than a cerebellar ataxia.

Syndrome of Inappropriate ADH Secretion

Hyponatremia is not uncommon in patients with GBS and, in some cases, has been shown to be accompanied by high urine osmolality and increased urinary sodium excretion, the essential features of syndrome of inappropriate

ADH secretion (SIADH). The mechanism for the production of this syndrome is obscure but hypothalamic involvement has been suggested. However, a more plausible explanation is that the increased ADH secretion is the result of neuropathy involving afferent fibers from vascular stretch receptors, that is, that the SIADH is a result of the autonomic neuropathy associated with GBS. In support of this hypothesis is the observation that experimental section of the vagus increases ADH secretion.

Pathological and Neuroimaging Abnormalities and Abnormalities of Central Conduction

From the foregoing, it is clear that there is little evidence to suggest that there is primary CNS involvement in most cases of GBS from a clinical point of view and it is certainly unnecessary to invoke primary CNS involvement to explain most of the clinical signs. However, there have been a number of reports of abnormal conduction in CNS pathways, abnormalities of computed tomography (CT) and MRI scans of the brain and even abnormal findings in pathological specimens that have led to the suggestion that the CNS is occasionally affected by the primary pathological process. In many of the patients described by Al-Din et al.,[64] some of whom probably had GBS, there was electrophysiological, radiological, or pathological evidence of CNS involvement. Of the 10 patients with areflexia and cranial nerve palsies, a picture most consistent with Miller-Fisher syndrome, there were five with significant alteration of level of consciousness at the outset, one of whom had seizures. In most, these clinical abnormalities occurred very early, perhaps reflecting persistent encephalitis related to the prodromal viral illness. Five patients also had abnormal CT scans, showing low density lesions in the brain stem, sometimes with contrast enhancement, and two patients had abnormal conduction in the central components of their brain stem auditory evoked potentials. Finally, one patient died after a protracted course and, at autopsy, had multiple foci of necrosis, gliosis, and inflammation in the brain stem without evidence of primary demyelination. However, these pathological changes may have been related to the prolonged illness. All of these patients had signs of CNS involvement early in the course of their neurological disease and none had significant peripheral or axial weakness, making it unlikely that the CNS signs could be attributed to metabolic disorders secondary to neuropathy. It is perhaps more likely that the CNS signs were manifestations of a viral encephalitis and that the GBS was the postinfectious manifestation of that same primary infection. Several other investigators have reported abnormalities of central conduction and neuroimaging in isolated cases whereas an equal number have sought, but failed to find, such abnormalities (reviewed in the section on Miller-Fisher syndrome, earlier in this chapter).

Most pathological studies have revealed little in the way of CNS involvement. Frequently, there is central chromatolysis, degeneration of central projections of peripheral axons, and occasional small perivascular foci of inflammatory cells. There have been occasional reports of cerebral edema. In most cases, there is no evidence that CNS demyelination occurs. However, inflammatory, macrophage-mediated demyelination of the CNS has occasionally been described in rare patients dying during the acute phase of the illness.[106,107]

With the numerous conflicting reports concerning CNS involvement in GBS it is difficult to determine with certainty the contribution of CNS injury to the symptoms and signs of GBS. However, it is safe to say that the CNS is only rarely involved and that the mechanism of involvement is unlikely to be immune-mediated demyelination. Furthermore, the clinical manifestations of any CNS involvement are trivial and do not contribute significantly to morbidity or mortality. Whenever symptoms and signs of CNS involvement are detected it is much more important to consider alternative explanations, such as hypoxia, sepsis, or hyponatremia, rather than attribute them to the GBS directly.

CNS Involvement in Chronic Inflammatory Demyelinating Polyradiculoneuropathy

The coexistence of central and peripheral demyelination is on a much firmer footing in chronic inflammatory demyelinating polyradiculoneuropathy (CIDP). Patients with clinically definite multiple sclerosis may have electrophysiological[109] and morphological[110] evidence of peripheral nerve involvement, although it is of little clinical consequence. More commonly, patients with CIDP have evidence of central demyelination on clinical, electrophysiological, CT, and MRI grounds.[111–115] In most cases, the central demyelination has little clinical impact, being apparent only on the sensitive MRI studies, although the group of patients described by Thomas et al.[114] had a clinical syndrome highly characteristic of multiple sclerosis. Feasby et al.[116] found that CNS lesions on MRI scans were limited to older patients in whom high signal lesions in the subcortical white matter are a common incidental finding. They suggest that these lesions may be ischemic, rather than a manifestation of coexistent central and peripheral demyelination.

Temporal Profile in GBS

GBS is an acute, monophasic neuropathy. In those cases in which there is a recognizable prodromal illness, neurological symptoms appear within 2 weeks in most patients. The earliest symptoms of pain and paresthesiae are followed within 24 to 48 hr by the onset of weakness. Often there are no sentinel sensory symptoms and the first complaint is weakness, which usually appears in the distal limb muscles but may occasionally affect proximal, truncal (including respiratory), or cranial musculature first. Rarely, symptoms of autonomic failure are the first to appear. Symptoms spread and progress over days to weeks and a nadir is reached within 1 week of the first symptom in approximately 50% of cases, within 2 weeks in 80%, and within 3 weeks in more than 90%. Recovery usually begins within 2 to 4 weeks after the nadir is reached, but may occasionally be delayed for months. The tempo of recovery is variable and depends largely on the degree of associated axonal degeneration. Recovery typically occurs over 3 to 6 months and more than 80% of patients make a complete functional recovery. The remainder have some deficits and about 5% of patients have a significant, permanent disability. Many clinical, electrophysiological, and laboratory features have been studied, early in the course of the disease, to determine whether they can accurately predict ultimate outcome. Only the electrophysiological examination has regularly provided useful prognostic information. If motor nerves are inexcitable or of very low amplitude (<10% of lower limit of normal) during the first week of illness, the prognosis is ominous. Similarly, needle EMG performed 3 to 4 weeks after the onset of the neurological symptoms will provide an estimate of the degree of associated axonal degeneration which, at least in some studies, correlated with ultimate outcome. It is important to emphasize that earlier EMG examination will likely underestimate the degree of associated axonal degeneration since spontaneous activity takes from 1 to 3 weeks to appear after axons are injured.

Exacerbations are uncommon in GBS, occurring in about 5% of cases. Once the recovery phase has begun, progressive improvement is to be expected. Some variation in the rate of recovery may be seen but unequivocal relapse should raise the suspicion of chronic relapsing neuropathy. This related disorder may present with a clinical and laboratory picture indistinguishable from GBS,[117] although usually the evolution is somewhat slower. However, it is distinguished from GBS by its tendency to relapse and slowly deteriorate over many years in a way analogous to multiple sclerosis. There have been several recent reports of an increased tendency for relapse to occur in otherwise typical GBS treated with plasmapheresis (see Chapter 6). However, neither the North American or French multicenter cooperative studies of plasmapheresis in GBS found any increase in the relapse rate when treated and untreated patients were compared. In those cases in which relapse was thought to be related to cessation of plasmapheresis, the relapse responded equally well to repeat plasmapheresis.

Summary

The classical clinical features of GBS are readily recognizable and provide little in the way of diagnostic confusion. However, atypical or restricted forms of the disease often occur, at least at the outset. With the development of treatment, which is most effective when applied early, recognition of these atypical and restricted patterns of disease have become much more important. With the improvements in respiratory care in paralyzed patients there has been a relative increase in morbidity and mortality due to autonomic instability, a generally underappreciated aspect of GBS. The complications of autonomic instability are not confined to patients with severe paralysis, and close observation in an intensive care unit if necessary is imperative in all GBS patients.

References

1. Landry O. Note sur la paralysie ascendante aigue. *Gaz Hebd Med*. 1859;6:472–474, 486–488.
2. Guillain G, Barré JA, Strohl A. Sur un syndrome de radiculo-nevrite avec hyperalbuminose du liquide cephalo-rachidien sans reaction cellulaire. Remarques sur les caracteres cliniques et graphique des reflexes tendineux. *Bull Mem Soc Med Hop Paris*. 1916;40:1462–1470.
3. Albers JW, Kelly JJ. Acquired inflammatory demyelinating polyneuropathies: clinical and electrodiagnostic features. *Muscle Nerve*. 1989;12:435–451.
4. Andersson T, Siden A. A clinical study of the Guillain-Barré syndrome. *Acta Neurol Scand*. 1982;66:316–327.
5. England JD. Guillain-Barré syndrome. *Annu Rev Med*. 1990;41:1–6.
6. Loffel NB, Rossi LN, Mumenthaler M, Lutschg J, Ludin H-P. The Landry-Guillain-Barré syndrome. Complications, prognosis and natural history in 123 cases. *J Neurol Sci*. 1977;33:71–79.
7. Marshall J. The Landry-Guillain-Barré syndrome. *Brain*. 1963;86:55–66.
8. Ravn H. The Landry-Guillain-Barré syndrome. A survey and a clinical report of 127 cases. *Acta Neurol Scand*. 1967;43(suppl 30):6–64.
9. Wiederholt WC, Mulder DW, Lambert EH. The Landry-Guillain-Barré-Strohl syndrome or polyradiculoneuropathy: historical review, report on 97 patients, and present concepts. *Mayo Clin Proc*. 1964;39:427–451.
10. Ropper AH, Shahani BT. Diagnosis and management of areflexic paralysis with emphasis on Guillain-Barré syndrome. In: Asbury AK, Gilliatt RW, eds. *Peripheral nerve disorders*. London: Butterworth;1984:21–45.
11. Mateer JE, Gutmann L, McComas CF. Myokymia in Guillain-Barré syndrome. *Neurology*. 1983;33:374–376.
12. Wasserstrom WR, Starr A. Facial myokymia in the Guillain-Barré syndrome. *Arch Neurol*. 1977;34:576–577.
13. Daube JR, Kelly JJ Jr, Martin RA. Facial myokymia with polyradiculoneuropathy. *Neurology*. 1979;29:662–669.
14. Albers JW, Allen AA, Bastron JA, Daube JR. Limb myokymia. *Muscle Nerve*. 1981;4:494–504.
15. Gutmann L. AAEM minimonograph #37: facial and limb myokymia. *Muscle Nerve*. 1991;14:1043–1049.
16. Preston DC, Kelly JJ. "Pseudospasticity" in Guillain-Barré syndrome. *Neurology*. 1991;41:131–134.
17. Winer JB, Hughes RAC, Osmond C. A prospective study of acute idiopathic neuropathy. I. Clinical features and their prognostic value. *J Neurol Neurosurg Psychiatry*. 1988;51:605–612.
18. Carrol WM, Mastaglia FL. "Locked-in coma" in postinfective polyneuropathy. *Arch Neurol*. 1979;36:46–47.
19. Loeb C, Mancardi GL, Tabaton M. Locked-in syndrome in acute inflammatory polyradiculoneuropathy. *Eur Neurol*. 1984;23:137–140.
20. Ropper AH. Severe acute Guillain-Barré syndrome. *Neurology*. 1986;429–432.
21. Haymaker W, Kernohan JW. The Landry-Guillain-Barré syndrome. A clinicopathologic report of fifty fatal cases and a critique of the literature. *Medicine*. 1949;28:59–141.
22. Eiben RM, Gersony WM. Recognition, prognosis and treatment of the Guillain-Barré syndrome (acute idiopathic polyneuritis). *Med Clin North Am*. 1963;47:1294–1306.
23. Ropper AH, Shahani BT. Pain in the Guillain-Barré syndrome. *Arch Neurol*. 1984;41:511–514.
24. Asbury AK, Fields HL. Pain due to peripheral nerve damage: an hypothesis. *Neurology*. 1984;34:1587–1590.
25. Calvin WH, Devor M, Howe JF. Can neuralgias arise from minor demyelination? Sponta-

neous firing, mechanosensitivity, and afterdischarge from conducting axons. *Exp Neurol.* 1982;75:755–763.

26. Dawson DM, Samuels MA, Morris J. Sensory form of acute polyneuritis. *Neurology.* 1988;38:1728–1731.
27. McLeod JG, Walsh JC, Prineas JW, Pollard JD. Acute idiopathic polyneuritis: a clinical and electrophysiological followup study. *J Neurol Sci.* 1976;27:145–162.
28. Osler W. *The principles and practice of medicine.* Edinburgh–London: Young J Pentland; 1892.
29. Tuck RR, McLeod JG. Autonomic dysfunction in Guillain-Barré syndrome. *J Neurol Neurosurg Psychiatry.* 1981;44:983–990.
30. Winer JB, Hughes RAC. Identification of patients at risk of arrhythmia in the Guillain-Barré syndrome. *Q J Med.* 1988;68:735–739.
31. Lichtenfeld P. Autonomic dysfunction in the Guillain-Barré syndrome. *Am J Med.* 1971;50:772–780.
32. Truax BT. Autonomic disturbances in the Guillain-Barré syndrome. *Semin Neurol.* 1984;4:462–468.
33. Appenzeller O, Marshall J. Vasomotor disturbance in Landry-Guillain-Barré syndrome. *Arch Neurol.* 1963;9:368–372.
34. Birchfield RI, Shaw C-M. Postural hypotension in the Guillain-Barré syndrome. *Arch Neurol.* 1964;10:149–157.
35. Davies AG, Dingle HR. Observations on cardiovascular and neuroendocrine disturbance in the Guillain-Barré syndrome. *J Neurol Neurosurg Psychiatry.* 1972;35:176–179.
36. Mitchell PL, Meilman E. The mechanism of hypertension in the Guillain-Barré syndrome. *Am J Med.* 1967;42:986–995.
37. Ahmad J, Kham AS, Siddigui MA. Estimation of plasma and urinary catecholamines in Guillain-Barré syndrome. *Jpn J Med.* 1985;24:24–29.
38. Saxenhofer H, Weidman P, Shaw S, Sulzer M, Siegrist P, Staubli M. Atrial natriuretic factor in the Landry-Guillain-Barré syndrome. *N Engl J Med.* 1988;319:448.
39. Wijdicks EFM, Ropper AH, Nathanson JA. Atrial natriuretic factor and blood pressure fluctuations in Guillain-Barré syndrome. *Ann Neurol.* 1990;27:337–338.
40. Laufer J, Passwell J, Keren G, Brandt N, Cohen BE. Raised plasma renin activity in the hypertension of the Guillain-Barré syndrome. *Br Med J.* 1981;282:1272–1273.
41. Hodson AK, Hurwitz BJ, Albrecht R. Dysautonomia in Guillain-Barré syndrome with dorsal root ganglioneuropathy, Wallerian degeneration and fatal myocarditis. *Ann Neurol.* 1984;15:88–95.
42. Frison JC, Sanchez L, Garnacho A, Bofill J, Olivero R, Miquel C. Heart rate variations in the Guillain-Barré syndrome. *Br Med J.* 1980;281:649.
43. Persson A, Solders G. R-R variations in Guillain-Barré syndrome: a test of autonomic dysfunction. *Acta Neurol Scand.* 1983;67:294–300.
44. Greenland P, Griggs RC. Arrhythmic complications in the Guillain-Barré syndrome. *Arch Intern Med.* 1980;140:1053–1055.
45. Favre H, Foex P, Guggisberg M. Use of demand pacemaker in a case of Guillain-Barré syndrome. *Lancet.* 1970;1:1062–1063.
46. Stewart IM. Arrhythmias in the Guillain-Barré syndrome. *Lancet.* 1973;1:665–666.
47. Emmons PR, Blume WT, DuShane JW. Cardiac monitoring and demand pacemaker in Guillain-Barré syndrome. *Arch Neurol.* 1975;32:59–61.
48. Maytal J, Eviatar L, Brunson SC, Gootman N. Use of demand pacemaker in children with Guillain-Barré syndrome and cardiac arrhythmias. *Pediatr Neurol.* 1989;5:303–305.
49. Palferman TG, Wright I, Doyle DV. Electrocardiographic abnormalities and autonomic dysfunction in Guillain-Barré syndrome. *Br Med J.* 1982;284:1231–1232.
50. Fergusson RJ, Wright DJ, Willey RF, Crompton GK, Grant IWB. Suxamethonium is dangerous in polyneuropathy. *Br Med J.* 1981;282:298–299.
51. Posner JB, Ertel NH, Kossmann RJ, Scheinberg LC. Hyponatremia in acute polyneuropathy. Four cases with the syndrome of inappropriate secretion of antidiuretic hormone. *Arch Neurol.* 1967;17:530–541.
52. Penney MD, Murphy D, Walters G. Resetting of osmoreceptor response as a cause of hyponatremia in acute idiopathic polyneuritis. *Br Med J.* 1979;2:1474–1476.
53. Pessin MS. Transient diabetes insipidus in the Landry-Guillain-Barré syndrome. *Arch Neurol.* 1972;27:85–86.
54. Fisher M. An unusual variant of acute idiopathic polyneuritis (syndrome of ophthalmoplegia, ataxia and areflexia). *N Engl J Med.* 1956;255:57–65.

55. Collier J. Peripheral neuritis. *Edinburgh Med J.* 1932;39:601–608, 672–713.
56. van Bogaert L, Maere M. Les polyradiculonevrites craniennes bilaterales avec dissociation albuminocytologique: formes craniennes des polyradiculonevrites du type Guillain et Barré. *J Belge Neurol Psychiatrie.* 1938;38:275–281.
57. Gibberd FB. Ophthalmoplegia in acute polyneuritis. *Arch Neurol.* 1970;23:161–164.
58. Elizan TS, Spire JP, Andiman RM, Baughman FA, Lloyd-Smith DL. Syndrome of acute idiopathic ophthalmoplegia with ataxia and areflexia. *Neurology.* 1971;21:281–292.
59. Davis MJ. A Guillain-Barré variant: ophthalmoplegia, ataxia and areflexia. *Mt Sinai J Med.* 1975;42:167–172.
60. Bell W, Van Allen M, Blackman J. Fisher syndrome in childhood. *Dev Med Child Neurol.* 1970;12:758–766.
61. Price RL, O'Connor PS, Rothner AD. Acute ophthalmoplegia, ataxia and areflexia (Fisher syndrome) in childhood. *Cleve Clin Q.* 1978;45:247–252.
62. Blau I, Casson I, Lieberman A, Weiss E. The not-so-benign Miller Fisher syndrome. A variant of the Guillain-Barré syndrome. *Arch Neurol.* 1980;37:384–385.
63. Littlewood R, Bajada S. Successful plasmapheresis in the Miller-Fisher syndrome. *Br Med J.* 1981;282:778–780.
64. Al-Din AM, Anderson M, Bickerstaff ER, Harvey I. Brainstem encephalitis and the syndrome of Miller Fisher. A clinical study. *Brain.* 1982;105:481–495.
65. Meienberg O, Ryffel E. Supranuclear eye movement disorders in Fisher's syndrome of ophthalmoplegia, ataxia and reflexia. Report of a case and literature review. *Arch Neurol.* 1983;40:402–405.
66. Jampel RS, Haidt SJ. Bell's phenomenon and acute idiopathic polyneuritis. *Am J Ophthal.* 1972;74:145–153.
67. Derakshan I, Loftj J, Kaufman B. Ophthalmoplegia, ataxia and hyporeflexia (Fisher's syndrome) with a midbrain lesion demonstrated by CT scanning. *Eur Neurol.* 1979;18: 361–366.
68. Barontini F, Sita D. The nosologic position of Fisher's syndrome (ophthalmoplegia, ataxia, areflexia). *J Neurol.* 1983;229:33–34.
69. Rudolph SH, Montensinos C, Shanzer S. Abnormal brainstem auditory evoked potentials in Fisher syndrome. *Neurology.* 1985;35(suppl 1):70.
70. Ropper AH, Shahani B. Proposed mechanism of ataxia in Fisher's syndrome. *Arch Neurol.* 1983;40:537–538.
71. Ropper AH. The CNS in Guillain-Barré syndrome. *Arch Neurol.* 1983;40:397–398.
72. Sauron B, Bouche P, Cathala H-P, Chain F, Castaigne P. Miller Fisher syndrome: clinical and electrophysiologic evidence of peripheral origin in 10 cases. *Neurology.* 1984;34:953–956.
73. Jamal GA, Ballantyne JP. The localization of the lesion in patients with acute ophthalmoplegia, ataxia and areflexia (Miller Fisher syndrome). A serial multimodal neurophysiological study. *Brain.* 1988;111:95–114.
74. Landau WM, Glenn C, Dust G. MRI in Miller Fisher variant of Guillain-Barré syndrome. *Neurology.* 1987;37:1431.
75. Ropper AH. Three patients with Fisher's syndrome and normal MRI. *Neurology.* 1988; 38:1630–1631.
76. Phillips MS, Stewart S, Anderson JR. Neuropathological findings in Miller Fisher syndrome. *J Neurol Neurosurg Psychiatry.* 1984;47:492–495.
77. Dehaene I, Martin JJ, Geens K, Cras P. Guillain-Barré syndrome with ophthalmoplegia: clinicopathologic study of the central and peripheral nervous systems, including the oculomotor nerves. *Neurology.* 1986;36:851–854.
78. Fross RD, Daube JR. Neuropathy in the Miller Fisher syndrome: clinical and electrophysiologic findings. *Neurology.* 1987;37:1493–1498.
79. Kaplan JG, Schaumburg HH, Sumner A. Relapsing ophthalmoparesis-sensory neuropathy syndrome. *Neurology.* 1985;35:595–596.
80. Donaghy M, Earl CJ. Ocular palsy preceding chronic relapsing polyneuropathy by several weeks. *Ann Neurol.* 1985;17:49–50.
81. Pellegrino-Levy. Contribution a l'etude de la paralysie ascendante aigue ou extenso-progressive aigue. *Arch Gen Med 6e Serie.* 1865;1:129–147.
82. Nelson KR, Gilmore RL, Massey A. Acoustic nerve conduction abnormalities in Guillain-Barré syndrome. *Neurology.* 1988;38:1263–1266.
83. Feasby TE, Gilbert JJ, Brown WF, et al. An acute axonal form of Guillain-Barré polyneuropathy. *Brain.* 1986;109:1115–1126.

84. Miller RG, Peterson C, Rosenberg NL. Electrophysiologic evidence of severe distal nerve segment pathology in the Guillain-Barré syndrome. *Muscle Nerve.* 1987;10:524–529.
85. Vallat JM, Hugon J, Tabaraud F, Leboutet MJ, Chazot F, Dumas M. Quatre cas de syndrome de Guillain-Barré avec lesions axonales. *Rev Neurol.* 1990;146:420–422.
86. Peterman AF, Daly PD, Dion FR. Infectious neuronitis (syndrome of Guillain-Barré) in children. *Neurology.* 1959;9:533–539.
87. Denny-Brown DE. The changing pattern of neurologic medicine. *N Engl J Med.* 1952; 246:839–846.
88. Gardner WJ, Spitler DK, Whitten C. Increased intracranial pressure caused by increased protein content in the cerebrospinal fluid; explanation of papilledema in certain cases of small intracranial and intraspinal tumors and in Guillain-Barré syndrome. *N Engl J Med.* 1954;250:932–936.
89. Morley JB, Reynolds EH. Papilloedema and the Landry-Guillain-Barré syndrome. Case reports and a review. *Brain.* 1966;89:205–222.
90. Weiss GB, Bajwa ZH, Mehler MF. Co-occurrence of pseudotumor cerebri and Guillain-Barré syndrome in an adult. *Neurology.* 1991;41:603–604.
91. Sullivan RL, Reeves AG. Normal cerebrospinal fluid protein, increased intracranial pressure and the Guillain-Barré syndrome. *Ann Neurol.* 1977;1:108–109.
92. Reid AC, Draper IT. Pathogenesis of papilloedema and raised intracranial pressure in Guillain-Barré syndrome. *Br Med J.* 1980;281:1393–1394.
93. Ropper AH, Marmarou A. Mechanism of pseudotumor in Guillain-Barré syndrome. *Arch Neurol.* 1984;41:259–261.
94. Joynt RJ. Mechanism of production of papilledema in the Guillain-Barré syndrome. *Neurology.* 1958;8:8–12.
95. Nikoskelainen E, Riekkinen P. Retrobulbar neuritis as an early symptom of Guillain-Barré syndrome. Report of a case. *Acta Ophthal.* 1972;50:111–115.
96. Behan PO, Lessell S, Roche M. Optic neuritis in the Landry-Guillain-Barré-Strohl syndrome. *Br J Ophthal.* 1976;60:5859.
97. Pall HS, Williams AC. Subacute polyradiculopathy with optic and auditory nerve involvement. *Arch Neurol.* 1987;44:88–887.
98. Toshwinal P. Demyelinating optic neuropathy with Miller-Fisher syndrome: the case for overlap syndromes with central and peripheral demyelination. *J Neurol.* 1987;234: 353–358.
99. Phanthumchinda K, Intragumtornchai T, Kasantikul V. Guillain-Barré syndrome and optic neuropathy in acute leukemia. *Neurology.* 1988; 38:1324–1326.
100. Uncini A, Treviso M, Basciani A, Onofrj M, Gambi D. Associated central and peripheral demyelination: an electrophysiological study. *J Neurol.* 1988;235:238–240.
101. Blennow G, Gamstorp I, Rosenberg R. Encephalomyeloradiculoneuropathy. *Dev Med Child Neurol.* 1968; 10:485–490.
102. Gamstorp I. Encephalomyeloradiculoneuropathy: involvement of the CNS in children with Guillain-Barré-Strohl syndrome. *Dev Med Child Neurol.* 1974;16:654–658.
103. Paulson GW. The Landry-Guillain-Barré-Strohl syndrome in childhood. *Dev Med Child Neurol.* 1970;12:604–607.
104. Willis J, Van den Bergh P. Cerebral involvement in children with acute and relapsing inflammatory polyneuropathy. *J Child Neurol.* 1988;3:200–204.
105. Amit R, Shapira Y, Blank A, Aker M. Acute, severe, central and peripheral nervous system combined demyelination. *Pediatr Neurol.* 1986;2:47–50.
106. Amit R, Glick B, Itzchak Y, Dgani Y, Meyer S. Acute severe combined demyelination. *Ann Neurol.* 1989;26:450. Abstract.
107. Lassmann H, Budka H, Schnaberth G. Inflammatory demyelinating polyradiculitis in a patient with multiple sclerosis. *Arch Neurol.* 1981;38:99–102.
108. Best PV. Acute polyradiculoneuritis associated with demyelinated plaques in the central nervous system. *Acta Neuropathol.* 1985;67:230–234.
109. Hopf HC, Eysholdt M. Impaired refractory periods of peripheral sensory nerves in multiple sclerosis. *Ann Neurol.* 1978;4:499–501.
110. Pollock M, Calder C, Allpress S. Peripheral nerve abnormality in multiple sclerosis. *Ann Neurol.* 1977;2:41–48.
111. Lewis RA, Sumner AJ, Brown MJ, Asbury AK. Multifocal demyelinating neuropathy with persistent conduction block. *Neurology.* 1982;32:958–964.
112. Mendell JR, Kolkin S, Kissel JT, Weiss KL, Chakeres DW, Rammohan KW. Evidence for

central system demyelination in chronic inflammatory demyelinating polyradiculo-neuropathy. *Neurology*. 1987;37:1291–1294.

113. Rubin M, Karpati G, Carpenter S. Combined central and peripheral myelinopathy. *Neurology*. 1987;37:1287–1290.

114. Thomas PK, Walker RWH, Rudge P, et al. Chronic demyelinating peripheral neuropathy associated with multifocal central nervous system demyelination. *Brain*. 1987;110:53–76.

115. Ohtake T, Komori T, Hirose K, Tanabe H. CNS involvement in Japanese patients with chronic inflammatory demyelinating polyradiculoneuropathy. *Acta Neurol Scand*. 1990; 81:108–112.

116. Feasby TE, Hahn AF, Koopman WJ, Lee DH. Central lesions in chronic inflammatory demyelinating polyneuropathy: an MRI study. *Neurology*. 1990;40:476–478.

117. Watson JDG, Spies JM, McLeod JG. Chronic inflammatory demyelinating polyneuropathy. A review of 74 patients. *Aust NZ J Med*. 1991;21(suppl 1):178. Abstract.

3

Diagnosis of Guillain-Barré Syndrome

The diagnosis of Guillain-Barré syndrome (GBS) is primarily clinical. The development of acute, areflexic paralysis with antecedent paresthesiae occurring 2 to 3 weeks after a febrile illness seldom presents a clinical dilemma. However, early in the course of the disease, when the clinical features are incompletely developed and with atypical clinical presentations, the diagnosis may be obscure. The cornerstone for the diagnosis is the electrodiagnostic evaluation, which can also provide objective data with which to follow the evolution of the disease, and invaluable prognostic information. Electrodiagnosis will be discussed in a subsequent chapter. When GBS is suspected clinically, the diagnosis can almost always be confirmed electrodiagnostically, supplemented by examination of the cerebrospinal fluid (CSF). The development of treatment with plasmapheresis, which is most effective when used early in the course of the disease, has made early diagnosis much more important.

Diagnostic Criteria

Controversy concerning the diagnostic criteria for GBS began almost as soon as the 1916 description of Guillain and his associates appeared.[1] Guillain, for many years, was of the opinion that fatality automatically excluded the diagnosis and was strident in his insistence on a distinction between Landry's paralysis, with its occasional mortality, and what he considered to be his

33

syndrome. Furthermore, he insisted that the CSF protein concentration was always above 300 mg/dl and was usually much higher and that the cell count could not exceed 10/mm[3]. Guillain published clinical criteria in 1936[2] (Table 3–1). In subsequent reports these criteria were periodically expanded and contracted depending on the prejudices of the authors. In 1960 Osler and Sidell[3] published restrictive criteria (Table 3–2) that served to stimulate a number of critical studies, specifically aimed at defining the syndrome more accurately.[4–9] In 1976, an epidemic consisting of more than a thousand GBS cases that followed the swine influenza vaccination program in the United States led to a colloquium sponsored by the National Institute of Neurological and Communicative Disorders and Stroke (NINCDS), which formulated a set of diagnostic criteria, first published in 1978 and now widely used.[10] These criteria were further modified in 1990, primarily by expanding the electro-diagnostic features.[11] However, without specific diagnostic markers for the disease, it must be emphasized that these criteria are no more than guidelines on which to base a reasonable diagnosis. The NINCDS diagnostic criteria are shown in Table 3–3 and the expanded electrodiagnostic criteria for de-myelination are shown in Table 3–4.

Table 3–1.   Guillain's Criteria (1936)

1. An onset characterized either by paralytic phenomena, paresthesiae, and/or pain, or all three, with or without premonitory symptoms such as sore throat, malaise, digestive disturbances, and stiffness of muscles.
2. Motor disturbances leading to flaccid paralysis of the lower limbs and later the trunk and upper limbs, the paralysis affecting chiefly the distal muscles of the limbs.
3. Fibrillary twitching, occasionally.
4. Slight atrophy of distal muscles, occasionally.
5. Ataxia in a moderate number.
6. Abolition of tendon reflexes in the domain of the paralyzed muscles and some-times beyond, and usually a preservation of the superficial reflexes, although as the disorder progresses they may be lost.
7. Subjective sensory disturbances such as pain, cramps, formication, and numb-ness.
8. Rather minor, infrequent, and transitory objective changes in sensibility, both cutaneous and deep, especially at the periphery of the limbs, and pain on application of pressure to muscles or to nerve trunks.
9. Astereognosis, occasionally.
10. Difficulty and slowness in micturition and loss of perception of the passage of urine in a few cases, and sphincter disturbances in even fewer.
11. Transient palsy of cranial nerves, notably the VIIth, and occasionally the extra-ocular nerves, the Vth, IXth, Xth, and XIIth, sometimes leading to fleeting disturbances of phonation, swallowing, respiration, and cardiac rhythm.

Table 3–2. Criteria of Osler and Sidell (1960)

1. The syndrome often, but not always, begins 1–3 weeks after an infection, most frequently a respiratory one. The exanthemas may be the precipitating cause, but if so there is always an interval between the illness and development of the syndrome.
2. The disease occurs at all ages and in both sexes, and the patient is afebrile when admitted to a hospital.
3. Dysesthesiae of the feet or hands or both usually precede the onset of paralysis.
4. There is a rapid onset of symmetrical loss of power, commonly in the proximal muscles of the legs and frequently in the proximal arm muscles. Sometimes, the distal muscles of the limbs are involved first. Severe involvement of the trunk muscles is uncommon. The word symmetrical signifies distribution and not necessarily degree. For example, one shoulder girdle may be weaker than the other, but if one is involved the other is too. Weakness usually spreads for some days after admission, seldom for more than 2 weeks.
5. The objective sensory loss is minimal and transient. Typically it varies, even during the same day. Any mode of sensation may be affected, but the most common finding is a fading "glove-and-stocking" hypesthesia and hypalgesia.
6. The bladder is never severely or directly involved, requiring repeated catheterization, but there may be transient difficulty in voiding, owing to immobility in bed and weakness of the abdominal muscles.
7. The tendon reflexes are lost or symmetrically diminished in milder cases.
8. The cranial nerves, most frequently the seventh, are often involved on one or both sides. We do not believe that the optic or auditory nerves are ever directly involved. Thus, we do not accept retrobulbar neuritis as part of the syndrome. When papilledema occurs it is late and has other causes than the primary disease.
9. Improvement begins usually before the third week, and continues without relapse.
10. The cerebrospinal fluid always shows a rise in protein content, without any marked rise in the number of cells, although this change may be delayed for a few days. A cell count over 10/mm³ should raise doubts of the diagnosis.
11. There is complete functional recovery, without residua, in 6 months. The degree of recovery is usually sufficient for discharge home in 3 months. The reflexes may remain reduced for a long time. Rarely, death from respiratory failure occurs in the early stages of the illness.
12. If examination or investigation reveals the presence of abnormalities other than those listed above, one should suspect another form of polyneuritis than the Guillain-Barré syndrome, or the presence of complicating disease that will alter the prognosis.

Diagnostic Laboratory Investigations

Because of the importance of electrodiagnostic studies in understanding the pathophysiology of demyelinating neuropathies as well as their critical role in establishing the diagnosis and determining prognosis in GBS, they will be described in a subsequent chapter (see Chapter 4). Only abnormalities of the CSF and blood will be discussed in this section.

Table 3–3.   NINCDS Criteria (1978)

Guillain-Barré syndrome is a recognizable entity for which the basis for diagnosis is descriptive in our present state of knowledge. The features that allow a diagnosis include clinical, laboratory, and electrodiagnostic criteria. The problem is not with recognition of a typical case, but with knowing the boundaries by which the core disorder is delimited. The following criteria are established, in light of current knowledge and opinion, to define those limits.

The presence of preceding events is frequent, but they are not essential to the diagnosis. Most commonly, preceding events are viral infections, but the association of Guillain-Barré syndrome with preceding surgery, inoculations, and mycoplasma infections is also known. In addition, Guillain-Barré syndrome occurs more frequently than by chance in the setting of preexisting illnesses such as Hodgkin's disease, lymphoma, or lupus erythematosus. Many patients with Guillain-Barré syndrome will have no history of any of these events, and the diagnosis should be made independent of them.

I. Features required for diagnosis
- A. Progressive motor weakness of more than one limb. The degree ranges from minimal weakness of the legs, with or without mild ataxia, to total paralysis of the muscles of all four extremities and the trunk, bulbar and facial paralysis, and external ophthalmoplegia.
- B. Areflexia (loss of tendon jerks). Universal areflexia is the rule, although distal areflexia with definite hyporeflexia of the biceps and knee jerks will suffice if other features are consistent.

II. Features strongly supportive of the diagnosis
- A. Clinical features (ranked in order of importance)
  1. *Progression.* Symptoms and signs of motor weakness develop rapidly but cease to progress by 4 weeks into the illness. Approximately 50% will reach the nadir by 2 weeks, 80% by 3 weeks, and more than 90% by 4 weeks.
  2. *Relative symmetry.* Symmetry is seldom absolute, but usually if one limb is affected the opposite is as well.
  3. *Mild sensory symptoms or signs.*
  4. *Cranial nerve involvement.* Facial weakness occurs in approximately 50% and is frequently bilateral. Other cranial nerves may be involved, particularly those innervating the tongue and muscles of deglutition, and sometimes the extraocular motor nerves. On occasion (less than 5%), the neuropathy may begin in the nerves to the extraocular muscles or other cranial nerves.
  5. *Recovery.* It usually begins 2–4 weeks after progression stops. Recovery may be delayed for months. Most patients recover functionally.
  6. *Autonomic dysfunction.* Tachycardia and other arrhythmias, postural hypotension, hypertension, and vasomotor symptoms, when present, support the diagnosis. These findings may fluctuate. Care must be exercised to exclude other bases for these symptoms, such as pulmonary embolism.
  7. *Absence of fever at the onset of neuritic symptoms.*

  Variants (not ranked)
  1. Fever at onset of neuritic symptoms.
  2. Severe sensory loss with pain.
  3. Progression beyond 4 weeks. Occasionally, a patient's disease will continue to progress for many weeks longer than 4 or the patient will have a minor relapse.

Table 3–3. (*Continued*)

    4. Cessation of progression without recovery or with major permanent residual deficit remaining.

    5. Sphincter function. Usually the sphincters are not affected, but transient bladder paralysis may occur during the evolution of symptoms.

    6. Central nervous system involvement. Ordinarily, Guillain-Barré syndrome is thought of as a disease of the peripheral nervous system. Evidence of central nervous system involvement is controversial. In occasional patients, such findings as severe ataxia interpretable as cerebellar in origin, dysarthria, extensor plantar responses, and ill-defined sensory levels are demonstrable, and these need not exclude the diagnosis if other features are typical.

  B. Cerebrospinal fluid features strongly supportive of the diagnosis

    1. CSF protein. After the first week of symptoms, CSF protein is elevated or has been shown to rise on serial lumbar punctures.

    2. CSF cells. Counts of 10 or fewer mononuclear leukocytes/mm^3 in CSF.

Variants

    1. No CSF protein rise in the period of 1–2 weeks after the onset of symptoms (rare).

    2. Counts of 11–50 mononuclear leukocytes/mm^3 in CSF.

  C. Electrodiagnostic features strongly supportive of the diagnosis

    Approximately 80% will have evidence of nerve conduction slowing or block at some point during the illness. Conduction velocity is usually less than 60% of normal, but the process is patchy and not all nerves are affected. Distal latencies may be increased to as much as 3 times normal. Use of F-wave responses often gives good indication of slowing over proximal portions of nerve trunks and roots. Up to 20% of patients will have normal conduction studies. Conduction studies may not become abnormal until several weeks into the illness.

III. Features casting doubt on the diagnosis

    1. Marked, persistent asymmetry of weakness.

    2. Persistent bladder or bowel dysfunction.

    3. Bladder or bowel dysfunction at onset.

    4. More than 50 mononuclear leukocytes/mm^3 in CSF.

    5. Presence of polymorphonuclear leukocytes in CSF.

    6. Sharp sensory level.

IV. Features that rule out the diagnosis

    1. A current history of hexacarbon abuse (volatile solvents; n-hexane and methyl n-butyl ketone). This includes huffing of paint lacquer vapors or addictive glue sniffing.

    2. Abnormal porphyrin metabolism indicating a diagnosis of acute intermittent porphyria. This would manifest as increased excretion of porphobilinogen and δ-aminolevulinic acid in the urine.

    3. A history of recent diphtheritic infection, either faucial or wound, with or without myocarditis.

    4. Features clinically consistent with lead neuropathy (upper limb weakness with prominent wrist drop; may be asymmetrical) and evidence of lead intoxication.

    5. The occurrence of a purely sensory syndrome.

    6. A definite diagnosis of a condition such as poliomyelitis, botulism, hysterical paralysis, or toxic neuropathy (e.g., from nitrofurantoin, dapsone, or organophosphorus compounds), which occasionally may be confused with Guillain-Barré syndrome.

**Table 3–4.   Proposed Electrodiagnostic Criteria
for Demyelination of Peripheral Nerve**

These criteria concern nerve conduction studies (including proximal nerve segments) in which the predominant process is demyelination.

Must have three of the following four features:

I.   Reduction in conduction velocity in two or more motor nerves.
   A.   <80% of lower limit of normal (LLN) if amplitude >80% of LLN.
   B.   <70% of LLN if amplitude <80% of LLN.
II.   Conduction block or abnormal temporal dispersion in one or more motor nerves: either peroneal nerve between ankle and below fibular head, median nerve between wrist and elbow, or ulnar nerve between wrist and below elbow.
   Criteria for partial conduction block:
   A.   <15% change in duration between proximal and distal sites and >20% drop in negative-peak area or peak-to-peak amplitude between proximal and distal sites.
   Criteria for abnormal temporal dispersion and possible conduction block:
   A.   >15% change in duration between proximal and distal sites and >20% drop in negative-peak area or peak-to-peak amplitude between proximal and distal sites.
III.   Prolonged distal latencies in two or more nerves.
   A.   >125% of upper limit or normal (ULN) if amplitude >80% of LLN.
   B.   >150% of ULN if amplitude <80% of LLN.
IV.   Absent F-waves or prolonged minimum F-wave latencies (10–15 trials) in two or more motor nerves.
   A.   >120% of ULN if amplitude >80% of LLN.
   B.   >150% of ULN if amplitude <80% of LLN.

CSF Examination

CSF PROTEIN CONCENTRATION

The current eponymous designation of this syndrome is primarily the result of the observation, reported by Guillain, Barré, and Strohl in 1916, that certain cases of acute paralysis with a good prognosis were associated with a very high CSF protein without an increase in cells (albuminocytologic dissociation). Queckenstedt[12] also noted this albuminocytologic dissociation in three cases of acute idiopathic neuropathy but the clinical features were insufficiently described to allow a certain diagnosis of GBS in his cases. The CSF picture, along with the uniformly good outcome, served to distinguish cases of GBS from poliomyelitis, the most common acute paralytic illness of the day. In the latter, CSF lymphocytic pleocytosis was the rule, sometimes exceeding 100 cells/ml, and CSF protein was only mildly elevated. Although variance from the original stringent definition is quite common, it still serves as a useful rule of thumb when evaluating patients with acute paralysis.

The increased CSF protein almost certainly predominantly reflects transudation of serum proteins into the CSF associated with an immunologically mediated attack on nerve roots as they traverse the subarachnoid space.[13,14]

The exact CSF protein concentration varies considerably from case to case, depending on the interval between onset of symptoms and lumbar puncture, the severity of disease, and the distribution of pathology. In cases in which the lumbar puncture is done within a few days of the onset of symptoms, the protein is often normal. In such cases a repeat examination should be done. In a study by Marshall,[4] the maximum elevation was seen between 4 and 18 days of the onset of the illness. McLeod et al.[15] found the CSF protein peaked between 10 and 20 days. Others have reported peak protein levels as late as 4 to 6 weeks after the onset of clinical symptoms.[16,17] Numerous other reports have attested to this general temporal sequence.[5,7,18–20] Cisternal CSF may have a normal protein concentration despite marked elevation of lumbar CSF protein,[13] supporting the concept that the protein in the CSF arises from spinal roots. Thus, the initial insistence by Guillain that, for a case to be considered an example of "his syndrome," the CSF protein concentration must be above 300 mg/dl and was usually above 1000 mg/dl, must be modified in light of subsequently accumulated evidence. Currently, the widely used NINCDS criteria do not require elevated CSF protein for the diagnosis, although the absence of an elevation is acknowledged as rare. Arnason[21] claims that as many as 20% of GBS cases have normal CSF protein throughout the course of the illness but most of the literature does not support this contention. For example, in seven large series published over several decades from different countries, totalling 570 apparently typical cases, only 9% did not have elevation of the CSF protein at some stage of the illness (Table 3–5). Furthermore, Marshall[4] found no case with normal CSF protein if more than one lumbar puncture was done.

In many patients, in keeping with the notion that GBS is an autoimmune disorder, there is an increase in the CSF concentration of gamma globulin,[22] often with oligoclonal bands.[23,24] Oligoclonal bands in the CSF without parallel bands in serum were reported by Link,[24] suggesting intrathecal gamma globulin synthesis. However, Spies et al.[25] found oligoclonal bands in the CSF in only 1 of 27 GBS patients and others have found oligoclonal bands

Table 3–5.   CSF Abnormalities

	% OF PATIENTS
CSF protein concentration*	
Elevated at initial spinal tap	86
Elevated at any time in illness	91
CSF cell count (/mm³)†	
< 5	68
5-10	20
11-20	7
> 20	5

*From seven series totaling 570 patients.[4,5,7,9,15,19,20]
†From four series totaling 301 patients.[4,5,7,15]

in both serum and CSF, challenging the notion of specific intrathecal synthesis.[21]

The elevation of CSF protein may be profound, sometimes exceeding 1500 mg/dl. It has been suggested that such high levels correlate with the development of intracranial hypertension and papilledema, occasionally seen in GBS, due to reduced CSF absorption through the arachnoid granulations into the vertex venous sinuses. However, the marked discrepancy between lumbar and cisternal CSF protein concentration, which would presumably be accentuated over the vertex, makes this hypothesis untenable. Furthermore, in 31 cases of intracranial hypertension associated with GBS reported by Morley and Reynolds[26] the CSF protein concentration was quite variable, being less than 200 mg/dl in eight cases.

CSF PLEOCYTOSIS

In 1936, Guillain stated "I refuse to recognize radiculoneuritis with hyperlymphocytosis or hypernucleosis as belonging to this syndrome." He conceded to a lymphocytic cell count as high as 10/mm[3] but not more. Although this finding is certainly the rule, some relaxation of such stringent criteria is necessary. The NINCDS criteria accept some cases with cell counts of 11 to 50/mm[3] but do not address the issue of the occasional higher counts. In cases in which the cell count is elevated above 10, there tends to be an inverse relationship between the number of cells and the CSF protein concentration.[15] In general, the highest cell counts have been reported early in the course of the disease when protein concentration tends to be low. This may reflect a persistent, low grade aseptic meningitis related to the preceding viral infection rather than a new inflammatory reaction associated with the developing radiculoneuropathy. However, Andersson and Siden[19] found both the highest protein concentration and cell counts in CSF taken 10 to 29 days after the onset of illness and CSF lymphocytosis exceeding 50 has been reported as many as 40 days after the onset of symptoms.[27] Marshall[4] found no change in the CSF cell count in seven patients who had two lumbar punctures whereas an eighth patient showed a rise in protein and a fall in cell count over the intervening 19 days. Overall, lymphocytic pleocytosis was present in more than 30% of 301 patients with otherwise typical GBS who were seen in the years before human immunodeficiency virus made its appearance and 5% of patients had cell counts greater than 20/mm[3] (Table 3–5).

Occasional CSF pleocytosis should not be surprising. Many of the early authors were sufficiently impressed with the clinical signs of meningeal irritation to use the term "meningoradiculitis" and felt that even intense CSF lymphocytosis did not exclude the diagnosis of GBS.[28–30] However, as Guillain firmly believed, many of these cases may not have been true GBS. The relatively frequent occurrence of GBS associated with cytomegalovirus and Epstein-Barr virus, notoriously chronic viral infections capable of causing a mild aseptic meningitis, may also contribute to the occasional cases with persistent lymphocytosis. In GBS associated with HIV infection, CSF pleocytosis is the rule; Cornblath et al.[31] have suggested that all cases of GBS with CSF pleocytosis should be tested for the presence of HIV antibodies. Similarly, there is usually a CSF pleocytosis in GBS in patients infected with *Borrelia burgdorferi* (Lyme disease).[32]

In cases with CSF lymphocytic pleocytosis, T lymphocytes predominate in the CSF, even though the peripheral blood T-lymphocyte count is usually reduced.[33,34]

Blood Testing

A number of abnormalities of the blood have been reported in GBS but none has diagnostic utility. There is often a moderate polymorphonuclear leukocytosis with an increase in the proportion of immature types while the lymphocyte count is often mildly reduced, especially during the earliest stages of the disease. The mild lymphopenia predominantly affects T lymphocytes but B lymphocytes may be increased.[33-36] Later in the course of the disease there may be a lymphocytosis. The erythrocyte sedimentation rate may also be increased. These findings are all nonspecific and may reflect the preceding viral infection rather than the postinfectious neuropathy.

In keeping with its immunological etiology, a wide variety of abnormalities of humoral and cell-mediated immunity have been described, but none is sufficiently specific to be diagnostically helpful. For example, Latov et al.[37] found peripheral nerve myelin antibodies in only 3 of 11 patients with GBS and others have reported similar results.[38-41] However, Koski et al.,[42] using a more sensitive assay, found antibodies in all 18 GBS patients whom they tested. Furthermore, they found a close correlation between antibody titer and the clinical stage of the disease; the titer was always highest early in the course and fell as progression stopped. In some patients, low titers of antibody persisted for months after the start of the clinical illness. In a search for specific antibodies, Ilyas et al.[43,44] reported IgM, IgA, or IgG antibodies to gangliosides in 5 of 26 patients with GBS. There was no consistency in the type of antibody; one patient reacted with GM1, two with GD1b, and two with both GD1a and GT1b, all of which are gangliosides found in peripheral nerve myelin. The antibody titers fell coincident with clinical improvement. These same antibodies were not found in control sera from normal individuals or from patients with other neurological diseases. Others have reported similar results.[45,46] The heterogeneity of these antiglycolipid antibody responses makes it unlikely that they have an important role in the pathogenesis of the disease.[47] Rostami et al.[48] searched for antibodies to galactocerebroside, which can produce acute, monophasic demyelination when injected into rat peripheral nerve, but could find none. In some patients, particularly those with rapidly progressing, severe disease, serum may produce demyelination when applied to tissue culture[49,50] or injected into the endoneurial compartment of a recipient animal.[51-54] However, although this phenomenon is important in understanding the pathogenesis of the disease, it is insufficiently sensitive to constitute a useful biological assay. In summary, whereas antibodies to a variety of the components of peripheral nerve myelin can be detected with some regularity in patients with GBS, serum antibody testing is neither sensitive nor specific enough to constitute a useful diagnostic method to assist in the diagnosis of clinically confusing cases. Nor is it certain that the antibodies that are seen are pathogenetic, rather than a nonspecific response to myelin damage.

Differential Diagnosis

GBS, in its classical form, seldom produces diagnostic confusion. However, unusual presentations may be mistaken for other disorders and occasionally other disorders are mistaken for GBS. The occasional difficulty in distinguishing GBS from other acute neuropathies is underscored in the report of Feit et al.,[55] who found alternative diagnoses in four out of six similar cases with acute neuropathy. Although a wide range of neurological disorders may have some features in common with GBS, this discussion will be confined to those that present acutely and that may occasionally be mistaken for GBS. Some of the disorders that may be mistaken for GBS are shown in Table 3–6.

Poliomyelitis and Other Acute Viral Anterior Horn Cell Diseases

GBS is now the most common cause of acute paralysis in the Western world. Poliomyelitis, the disease that previously laid claim to that dubious distinction, was the quintessential acute paralytic disease up until the 1950s, when large scale vaccination programs almost completely eliminated it from developed countries. Poliomyelitis remains a scourge in underdeveloped countries and occasional cases still occur in North America[56] and other developed countries, often in nonvaccinated individuals exposed to recently vaccinated

Table 3–6.   Disorders that May be Mistaken for GBS

Acute motor neuron diseases
Intoxications
Porphyric neuropathy
Vasculitic neuropathy
Neuromuscular junction diseases
Locked-in syndrome
CIDP with acute presentation
Acute sensory neuronopathy
Acute pandysautonomia
Acute transverse myelopathy
Hysteria

infants.[57–59] However, occasional infections with the wild virus also continue in developed countries; an outbreak of type 3 poliovirus infection occurred in Finland as recently as 1984.[60]

A host of other viruses, most commonly the enteroviruses, with a predilection for the anterior horn cell, constitute a more common cause of acute viral anterior myelopathy in developed countries[61] (Table 3–7). In addition, rabies infection can occasionally be largely confined to the spinal cord and cranial nerve nuclei, affecting the ventral and dorsal gray matter equally, and causing lower motor neuron paralysis with cranial nerve palsies that may superficially resemble GBS. However, rabies is much more commonly characterized by a severe, usually fatal, disseminated encephalomyelitis. Epidemic acute paralysis has been described in young people in China (the "China Syndrome"),[62] which is characterized physiologically and pathologically by motor neuron degeneration and may have a viral etiology, although no infectious agent has been identified.[63,64] Similar epidemic cases have been described in children in Mexico,[65] associated with noninflammatory chromatolysis of the anterior cells and some cases with argyrophilic degeneration of motor nuclei. The Mexican cases may represent a viral disorder, although some of the cases could have been due to ingestion of Buckthorn berries (see below). Rare sporadic cases of acute motor neuron disease with good prognosis for recovery have also been described in the United States and may have a viral etiology.[66,67]

The clinical features of poliovirus infection and of the other acute, viral infections of the anterior horn cell are essentially identical. Recognition that a suspected poliovirus infection is due to another virus is invariably retrospective, resulting from negative poliovirus culture and serological studies. The first sign of infection is generally a brief febrile illness, often a gastroenteritis, followed within 7 to 14 days by acute paralysis. Although the poliovirus is highly infectious, only a small proportion of infected individuals develop the paralytic phase. During poliovirus epidemics, serological studies suggest that less than 1% of infected individuals develop any symptoms of infection and only 30% to 60% of those develop a paralytic illness. The risk of developing paralysis varies with age; adults are more than 10 times as likely to develop paralysis.[68] After the initial febrile episode there is usually a temporary improvement, although in some cases progression to the neurological phase of the illness occurs immediately. The neurological illness

Table 3–7. Acute Motor Neuron Diseases

Poliomyelitis
Other viral anterior myelopathies (rabies, enteroviruses)
"China syndrome"
Cytoplasmic and nuclear neuronopathy
Sporadic idiopathic motor neuron disease

begins with a recurrence of systemic symptoms of fever, headache, and neck stiffness, sometimes accompanied by an alteration in mental status. However, these signs, which accompany invasion of the central nervous system by the virus, may be trivial or entirely lacking. Muscle pain, particularly in the back, and widespread fasciculations then appear, heralding the onset of flaccid paralysis, which may be focal or generalized, although it is usually asymmetrical. Atrophy develops rapidly over about a week. Exercise during the early phase of the neurological illness increases the severity of the paralysis, particularly in the region of the body that has been exercised. No anterior horn cell is completely immune from attack, with bulbar and phrenic involvement being the major causes of death. However, oculomotor involvement, as in other disorders of the anterior horn cell, is rare. Although the brunt of the injury is borne by the anterior horn cell, some bulbar and spinal long tract involvement may be seen, probably as a result of nonspecific injury related to inflammation and edema of nearby motor neurons, secondarily involving white matter. Thus, sensory symptoms are common and objective sensory loss has occasionally been reported.[69] Similarly, autonomic involvement,[70] nystagmus, and altered sensorium[71] occasionally are seen. Cases with sensory and autonomic signs and symptoms are particularly likely to be mistaken for GBS in developed countries. Conversely, GBS has been described after vaccination against poliovirus[72] and may be mistaken for vaccine-associated paralytic poliomyelitis. The illness reaches its nadir within 2 to 4 weeks and complete or partial functional recovery begins slowly thereafter. Vaccine-associated poliomyelitis tends to be less severe and may be diagnosed late or missed completely,[59] although severe paralysis may occur.[58]

Thus, with the occurrence of an acutely evolving paralysis, appearing 10 to 14 days after a gastroenteritis and sometimes associated with back pain and sensory and autonomic symptoms and signs, it is easy to understand why poliomyelitis might be mistaken for GBS, particularly in developed countries. Conversely, cases of GBS are undoubtedly occasionally missed in areas endemic for poliomyelitis.

CSF examination is the most critical investigation in patients with suspected viral anterior myelopathies. Although the CSF may occasionally be normal, there is usually a pleocytosis that is initially composed of both polymorphonuclear leukocytes and lymphocytes but that quickly becomes predominantly lymphocytic. This pleocytosis is usually less than 100 cells/mm³ but higher cell counts may be seen. CSF protein is normal but may be slightly increased and is only rarely as high as 200 mg/dl. This contrasts with the typical albuminocytologic dissociation of GBS.

Nerve conduction studies are also of critical importance in distinguishing between these two disorders. In poliomyelitis, the motor nerve conduction studies are characterized by low amplitude compound muscle action potentials (CMAPs) with normal or only slightly slowed nerve conduction velocity and insignificant prolongation of distal motor latency and F-wave latency. True conduction block does not occur and the motor responses are not dispersed. However, early in the evolution of the paralysis in poliomyelitis, motor responses may be elicitable with distal, but not proximal, stimulation in completely paralyzed muscles (pseudoblock) due to conduction continuing in motor axons undergoing wallerian degeneration. Sensory nerve conduction studies are normal in both conditions in the first few days but become abnormal after that in about 70% of patients with GBS. Fasciculations are often seen in poliomyelitis but are rare in GBS. Furthermore, in poliomyelitis there is prominent fibrillation in the weak muscles, usually appearing during the second and third weeks, and exceeding that seen in most cases of GBS.

Although each of the clinical, CSF, and electrodiagnostic features of poliomyelitis may be seen rarely in GBS, the combination of all of them in a single patient excludes the diagnosis. The diagnosis of suspected poliomyelitis can be confirmed by retrieving poliovirus from pharyngeal washings in the first few days of the illness or from stool samples for several weeks. Acute and convalescent sera can also be assayed for antibodies against poliovirus or other potential viral pathogens.

Biological Toxins

TICK PARALYSIS

Tick paralysis (see Table 3–8), as the name indicates, is an acute paralytic illness resulting from a salivary toxin injected while the tick is feeding on its host.[73-75] Paralysis can be transferred to animals by injection of homogenates of engorged ticks but the nature of the toxin remains obscure.[76,77] The clinical picture is similar to GBS and the diagnosis is unlikely to be made unless the tick is looked for and found. It is most often seen in children and is more common in girls. The tick is usually located on the scalp, concealed by the hair, and may be difficult to find without shaving the patient. Other sites include the auditory canal and the perianal area. Tick paralysis is seen in many geographic areas and with several different species of tick.[77,78] In North America, tick paralysis is most commonly seen in the northwestern United

Table 3–8. Acute Intoxications Affecting the Neuromuscular System

Biological toxins
  Tick paralysis
  Diphtheria
  Ciguatera
  Buckthorn
  Botulism
  Snake bite paralysis
Environmental toxins
  Heavy metals (arsenic, thallium, gold)
  Organophosphates
  Alcohol

States and in Canada; the most commonly associated tick is *Dermacentor andersoni*. However, cases have been reported from eastern and southern states and from the southern midwest. In Australia, another area from which tick paralysis is commonly reported, the offending tick is *Ixodes holocyclus*. Tick paralysis has also been seen in Africa and parts of Asia but not in Central or South America.

The neurologic syndrome generally begins 3 to 5 days after the tick has been attached. The earliest symptoms are often nonspecific with complaints of fatigue and irritability followed by paresthesiae and occasionally ataxia. Within a day or two a flaccid, areflexic paralysis develops, beginning distally and rapidly ascending over hours and often involving bulbar and respiratory muscles. Occasionally, the paralysis may be focal, in the region of attachment of the tick.[75] Sensory examination is normal. All of the neurologic manifestations rapidly resolve once the tick is completely removed. Failure of the patient to improve is usually due to incomplete removal of the tick or to a second, undetected tick.

Although in its fully developed form tick paralysis is strikingly similar to GBS, there are important differences that provide clues to the correct diagnosis. The brevity of the prodrome and the extraordinarily rapid evolution of the paralysis, which are characteristic of tick paralysis, are unusual in GBS. CSF protein is not elevated in tick paralysis but may also be normal early in the course of GBS. However, persistence of a normal CSF protein is unusual in GBS and should stimulate a search for alternative causes of paralysis. The electrodiagnostic studies are invaluable in distinguishing tick paralysis from GBS. The predominant abnormality is a striking reduction in the amplitude of the compound muscle action potential with negligible conduction slowing, although there is mild prolongation of the distal motor latency. Sensory nerve conduction studies are all within the normal range,[79,80] although serial studies after removal of the tick have shown progressive shortening of sensory latencies, indicating mild involvement of sensory axons as is suggested by the frequent occurrence of paresthesiae.[80] There is no demonstrable motor conduction block, although the low amplitude motor responses have been attributed to conduction block in terminal motor axons, at least in animals.[81] Routine studies of neuromuscular transmission are normal in humans but animal studies showed a defect in acetylcholine release from the presynaptic terminal.[82,83] These findings contrast dramatically with the usual findings in GBS, in which there is marked conduction slowing often with accompanying motor conduction block. However, early in the course of GBS, electrodiagnostic studies may be normal and in some cases, the only abnormality is a marked reduction in motor response amplitudes (see Chapter 4). IgE antibodies to specific ticks can be detected in individuals with a systemic reaction and have potential as an aid to diagnosis in endemic areas.[84] However, the accurate and timely diagnosis depends primarily on a high index of suspicion combined with a careful search for the tick.

DIPHTHERIA

Diphtheritic neuropathy has become rare in countries with established vaccination programs against diphtheria. It is an acute demyelinating neuropathy resulting from absorption of the toxin produced by the bacterium *Corynebacterium diphtheriae*, which produces a febrile tonsillitis and pharyngitis. Although it is extremely rare, it should be considered in any patient with an acute demyelinating neuropathy in whom there has been a history of preceding severe pharyngitis, even in the absence of a pharyngeal membrane. Typically, palatal weakness is the earliest sign, presumably reflecting local production of the neurotoxin.[85] This may be the only sign of the neuropathy but about half of the cases go on to develop a generalized neuropathy.[86] Other cranial nerves then become involved, often beginning with paralysis of accommodation.[87,88] Limb weakness follows but is less severe and typically affects the proximal muscles more than the distal ones.[85] Respiratory involvement rarely occurs.[85] There is usually areflexia, although the reflexes may be preserved early.[88,89] Sensory symptoms are common but objective sensory loss is usually trivial. Autonomic neuropathy is not usually seen. Sinus tachycardia is common[87] but probably is secondary to the toxic myocarditis that occurs and is the major cause of death. One important difference between diphtheritic neuropathy and GBS is the rate of evolution. In the former, the nadir of the weakness is usually delayed for as much as 3 months after the first sign of pharyngeal paralysis.

The CSF in diphtheritic neuropathy is identical to GBS, with an elevated protein without pleocytosis.[90] Similarly, the electrodiagnostic studies are those of an acute demyelinating neuropathy, identical to GBS.[89,91] As a result, the diagnosis of diphtheritic neuropathy rests on the recognition of the initial faucial involvement.

INGESTED MARINE TOXINS

Acute neurological disease may result from ingestion of a preformed neurotoxin produced by several varieties of marine animals.[92,93] Common to these closely related toxins (tetrodotoxin from pufferfish, ciguatoxin from ciguatera, saxitoxin from shellfish) is an ability to block the sodium channel. There are prominent paresthesiae, particularly in a perioral distribution, and sometimes pain. These sensations are accompanied by objective sensory loss. With pufferfish poisoning and ciguartera, the sensory symptoms are followed by paralysis, which is rarely severe but has, on occasion, involved the respiratory muscles. Autonomic features may be seen. Reflexes may be normal or depressed. CNS toxicity may also occur with ataxia, tremor, nystagmus, and visual loss. The neurological syndrome may be accompanied by vomiting and diarrhea. The clinical syndrome only superficially resembles GBS. Furthermore, the CSF is normal and nerve conductions are also normal[94] or show mild slowing, mainly involving sensory nerves.[95]

BUCKTHORN INTOXICATION

Buckthorn (Karwinskia humboldtiana) is a shrub that is found in parts of northern Mexico and the southwestern United States. Ingestion of its berries causes an acute predominantly demyelinating neuropathy in humans and domestic animals.[96] The neuropathy typically appears after a delay of 1 to 2 weeks and progresses rapidly, reaching a nadir within 2 to 3 days. It is a more quintessentially ascending paralysis than GBS, beginning in the feet and involving proximal limb and axial muscles later. Respiratory and cranial nerve involvement may occur and is the usual cause of death in fatal cases. Sensory loss is present but is overshadowed by the prominent paralysis: tendon reflexes are reduced or absent. Although spontaneous recovery occurs in most cases, it may be protracted and some permanent sequelae may be seen.[97]

The Hepatic Porphyrias

This group of rare, dominantly inherited disorders includes acute intermittent porphyria, variegate porphyria, and coproporphyria, all of which may be associated with neuropathy, the clinical features of which are identical.[98–100] The neuropathy is usually acute in onset and predominantly motor, including occasional involvement of the cranial nerves, and may be mistaken for GBS. There is usually some degree of areflexia, although ankle reflexes may be spared even when the patellar reflexes are lost. The accompanying autonomic instability with sphincter disturbances, marked tachycardia, and widely vacillating blood pressure serves to compound the confusion. Rather than being preceded by a febrile illness, porphyric neuropathy is characteristically ushered in by abdominal pain, constipation, vomiting, and often mental changes, although even these may be mistaken for a prodrome to GBS. Attacks are often precipitated by barbiturates and sometimes by other drugs. Accompanying changes in urine color, although not invariable, provide a valuable clue to the diagnosis. The weakness in porphyria is typically proximal and the arms may be more affected than the legs. This distribution is somewhat unusual for GBS but does not provide a reliable distinction. Sensory loss is unusual but if it occurs it may also be proximal whereas any sensory changes in GBS are distal, even when paralysis is proximally accentuated. Finally, in GBS there is almost always widespread reflex loss with early loss of the ankle jerk. Conversely, paradoxical preservation of the ankle reflexes in the face of absent patella reflexes is more commonly seen in porphyria. Although these are the most common features of porphyric neuropathy, it should be stressed that the presentation is extremely variable and clinical distinction from GBS may be difficult, if not impossible.

Distinction between GBS and porphyric neuropathy can almost always be made on electrophysiological grounds, if the diagnosis is suspected.[101] Nerve conduction studies in porphyric neuropathy typically show normal or slightly reduced amplitude motor responses with normal conduction velocity. Needle electromyography reveals signs of acute denervation (fibrillation potentials). These are the electrophysiological signs of axonal or neuronal degeneration, the usual pathology in porphyric neuropathy, rather than demyelination. However, even the electrophysiological manifestations of porphyric neuropathy are not constant or completely predictable. Carlson et al.[102] reported two patients with porphyria who developed a neuropathy that was clinically, electrophysiologically, and morphologically indistinguishable from GBS. Both patients presented with acute quadriparesis and fulfilled the NINCDS clinical criteria for the diagnosis of GBS. In addition, nerve conduction studies showed partial conduction block, reduced conduction velocity, prolonged distal motor latencies, and prolonged latency or absent F-waves, the characteristic electrodiagnostic findings of demyelination. Finally, one patient had inflammatory demyelination on the sural nerve biopsy. The patients slowly recovered over several months.

In porphyria, the CSF protein is usually normal, although slight elevation (up to 100 mg/dl) may occur. Diagnosis of porphyria can be confirmed by the presence of porphyrins or their precursors (porphobilinogen, delta-aminolevulinic acid) in the urine. These substances are present even when the urine is not discolored since urinary discoloration depends on the pH. Tests for the specific enzyme deficiency in blood cells are also now available.

Vasculitic Neuropathy

Neuropathy is a common complication of the systemic disorders in which vasculitis is a feature but it usually evolves in a subacute or chronic fashion.[103] Acute mononeuropathy multiplex, with a few individual nerves sequentially involved, may complicate systemic necrotizing vasculitis of the type seen in polyarteritis nodosa, Churg-Strauss syndrome, and occasionally in rheumatoid arthritis.[104] However, neither the slowly evolving neuropathy nor acute mononeuropathy multiplex is likely to be mistaken for GBS. Rarely, an acutely evolving neuropathy in which the multifocality is less obvious may occur in patients with necrotizing vasculitis and superficially resemble GBS.[103,105,106] Even in its most florid form, this neuropathy usually evolves more slowly than GBS. Pain is common and sensory and motor symptoms and signs occur with equal frequency. Reflexes are reduced or absent concordant with the severity of the other signs. Cranial nerve involvement is not common and respiratory failure is extremely rare. Patients usually appear ill, reflecting the underlying systemic disease, the sedimentation rate is often very high (>100 mm/hr), and there is other laboratory evidence of vasculitis. The CSF is usually normal, although modest elevation of the protein concentration may be seen. Electrophysiologically, vasculitic neuropathy does not resemble GBS.[104] Sensory and motor responses are reduced in amplitude or absent and conduction velocity, when it can be recorded, is normal or only slightly slowed. Conduction block and temporal dispersion, if they occur at all, must be very rare. True conduction block has been described in vasculitis neuropathy[107] but, in most cases, segmental amplitude changes simulating conduction block simply reflect temporarily continuing conduction in the distal segment of acutely infarcted peripheral nerves. The diagnosis of vasculitic neuropathy can usually be confirmed by nerve biopsy.[108] Thus, although systemic vasculitis may occasionally be complicated by an acute neuropathy, the resemblance to GBS is superficial and the disorders can easily be distinguished on clinical, electrophysiological, and laboratory grounds.

Neuromuscular Junction Disorders

Myasthenia gravis and botulism may occasionally present with apparently acute onset of paralysis. Similarly, the venom from several species of snake and some marine animals (e.g., sea urchin) may cause an acute paralytic illness by interfering with neuromuscular transmission at the pre- or post-synaptic level. Hypermagnesemia and intoxication with certain antibiotics (particularly aminoglycosides) may also cause weakness by interfering with neuromuscular transmission but almost always in patients with predisposing conditions such as myasthenia gravis. In all of these disorders (see Table 3–9) there is predominant involvement of the cranial nerves, particularly the extraocular muscles, and there is often internal ophthalmoplegia as well. There are no sensory symptoms or signs and reflexes are not lost in myasthenia gravis, although they are commonly depressed or absent in botulism and snake bite paralysis. CSF examination and nerve conduction studies are normal whereas repetitive stimulation studies confirm the presence of a neuromuscular transmission defect.

The Locked-in Syndrome

Acute infarction of the basis pontis may produce flaccid paralysis and bulbar palsy (the locked-in syndrome), which superficially resembles GBS.[109,110] In the acute phase, the reflexes may be depressed, rather than increased, but become increased with time, and plantar responses are usually extensor. Moreover, there is no history of preceding febrile illness and the evolution of the paralysis is much more rapid. CSF and electrodiagnostic studies are usually normal apart from abnormalities of the blink reflex.

Table 3–9.   Acute Neuromuscular Junction Disorders

Myasthenia gravis
Botulism
Hypermagnesemia
Snake bite paralysis
Antibiotic toxicity (aminoglycosides)

Acute Toxic Neuropathies

Most toxic peripheral neuropathies (Table 3–8) are not as acute in their pattern of evolution as GBS. However, the delayed neuropathies that result from acute intoxications may cause diagnostic confusion if the history of preceding exposure is not forthcoming.

HEAVY METALS

The most commonly seen heavy metal toxic neuropathy results from arsenic ingestion in either its organic or inorganic form.[111] A similar syndrome may be seen after acute thallium poisoning. Other heavy metal neuropathies evolve much more slowly and do not mimic GBS. Acute poisoning with arsenic or thallium can cause gastrointestinal symptoms that may be mistaken for a prodromal gastroenteritis.[112] These symptoms typically subside and are then followed, 2 to 3 weeks later, by acute, areflexic paralysis and paresthesiae or dysesthesiae. To compound the confusion, the CSF protein is often elevated without pleocytosis (albuminocytologic dissociation). Furthermore, electrodiagnostic studies may be similar. Acute toxic neuropathies are characterized predominantly by axonal degeneration but multifocal segmental conduction block may be transiently seen during the acute phase. Intoxications frequently involve other systems, particularly the CNS, but diagnosis depends on obtaining a history of exposure. Since this type of toxic neuropathy follows massive exposure by ingestion, rather than chronic low-level exposure, such a history is usually available. However, the possibility of concealed intentional ingestion (suicidal or homicidal) causing a delayed neuropathy of this type must be borne in mind.

Neuropathy may also complicate the treatment of rheumatoid arthritis with gold salts. Although it has been described as Guillain-Barré–like[113] the resemblance is superficial. The most commonly described neuropathy with gold therapy evolves in a subacute fashion, over weeks to months, and is characterized both morphologically and electrophysiologically by predominant axonal degeneration.[114] However, an acute neuropathy more akin to GBS has rarely been described, with slow nerve conduction velocity and typical albuminocytologic dissociation in the CSF.[115,116] Whether these rare occurrences represent more than a coincidental relationship to gold therapy is open to doubt.[117]

ORGANOPHOSPHATES

The other toxins that may cause an acute but delayed neuropathy after exposure are the organophosphate compounds. The immediate effects of exposure are related to the anticholinesterase properties of these compounds.[118,119] Intoxicated individuals develop gastrointestinal symptoms and muscle twitching proceeding to obtundation and seizures in the more severe cases. If the acute phase is survived, after a delay of days to weeks, an acute axonal neuropathy develops. The development of neuropathy is independent of the anticholinesterase properties and depends instead on suppression of the enzyme, neuropathy target esterase (NTE).[120] The onset of paralysis is preceded by sharp cramping pains in the legs and paresthesiae in the hands and feet. Weakness involves both proximal and distal muscles, and cranial nerves (particularly the oculomotor nerves) are involved in about half the cases.[119] Respiratory failure rarely occurs. Ankle reflexes are lost but other reflexes are usually normal, although complete areflexia has been described. Depending on the severity of the intoxication, recovery begins in 3 to 6 weeks and may be complete in mild cases. However, during the recovery phase, clinical signs of spinal long tracts emerge, having been masked by the neuropathy during the acute phase. Permanent spasticity and posterior column sensory loss are common in the more severely affected cases. Distinction from GBS depends mainly on obtaining a history of exposure and recognizing the acute cholinergic effects that precede the neuropathy. Clinically, sensory phenomena are more prominent and reflex loss is usually less in organophosphate neuropathy. Tissue cholinesterase and NTE levels are depressed early but have returned to normal by the time the neuropathy develops.[120] Electrodiagnostic studies show a pure axonal neuropathy and the spinal fluid is normal. Classical GBS has been described after organophosphate exposure but probably is coincidental.[121]

ACUTE ALCOHOLIC NEUROPATHY

An acutely evolving neuropathy, similar to GBS, has also been described in chronic alcoholics.[122,123] Tabaraud et al.[123] described eight patients with a severe neuropathy, superficially mimicking GBS, that was manifested as areflexic paralysis that evolved over 1 to 3 weeks. In six patients the weakness was primarily proximal and in three, artificial ventilation was required. The patients differed from GBS in several important respects. All had severe sensory loss, the CSF protein was invariably normal, and the electrodiagnostic and morphologic studies indicated severe axonal degeneration. These features in combination effectively exclude the diagnosis of GBS.

A plethora of other toxic agents has been implicated in the pathogenesis of an acute neuropathy akin to GBS. However, in the vast majority of toxic neuropathies the evolution is much slower and confusion with GBS is unlikely. Isolated case reports purporting to show a relationship between an acute neuropathy and a particular toxin are unconvincing.

Chronic Inflammatory Demyelinating Polyneuropathy

Occasionally, a neuropathy destined to run a chronic or relapsing course has an acute presentation. Watson et al.[124] reported that 16% of a group of CIDP patients had an acute onset and had received an initial diagnosis of GBS. In such cases there is no reliable way to distinguish between these two similar but distinct disorders since they are both multifocal demyelinating neuropathies that are presumed to be immunologically mediated. Usually, even in the most acute presentation of CIDP, the evolution is somewhat slower, reaching a nadir after 4 weeks. However, clinical features may be otherwise identical, CSF protein may be elevated, and the electrodiagnostic features are essentially identical. Distinction is of more than academic interest, since CIDP is steroid responsive whereas GBS is not. However, both disorders may respond to plasmapheresis, which has become almost routine treatment for GBS, so a delay in diagnosis is usually all that results.

Acute Sensory Neuronopathy

Although sensory symptoms may be prominent in GBS, objective sensory loss is usually trivial while weakness is almost invariably found. Conversely, in the syndrome of acute sensory neuronopathy, there are prominent sensory symptoms associated with objective sensory loss, usually predominantly affecting the functions subserved by the larger myelinated axons. Complaints of weakness are frequent, perhaps accounting for the sometime confusion with GBS. However, testing of strength in individual muscles reveals no objective weakness. The symptoms may occur after a febrile illness, usually appearing within a few days and are of acute onset and progression, reaching their nadir within a week.[125,126] Early reports suggested that this disorder might be a toxic neuronopathy, related to antibiotics, since the patients had received antibiotics for their preceding febrile illness.[125] The patients often complain of pain or a feeling of tightness, followed by widespread sensory loss that may involve the face and trunk as well as limbs, often in a patchy distribution. There is a prominent sensory ataxia as well as loss of cutaneous sensibility. There is usually complete areflexia. Prognosis for full recovery is gloomy; only 8 of the 42 patients described by Windebank et al.[126] recovered completely. However, 22 were able to carry out most of their premorbid activities, albeit with significant persistent sensory deficits. A subacute sensory neuronopathy, identical except for its rate of evolution, occurs as a paraneoplastic disorder, usually associated with oat cell carcinoma of the lung[127] and with Sjögren's syndrome.[128] In addition, a chronic sensory neuronopathy is seen in patients with pyridoxine intoxication.[129]

The CSF picture in acute sensory neuronopathy is variable but may mimic GBS by having elevated CSF protein without pleocytosis. In other cases there is a marked pleocytosis with normal protein. Electrodiagnostic studies are particularly useful in separating the two disorders. In sensory neuronopathy, sensory nerve action potentials are absent or of extremely reduced amplitude, with relatively preserved conduction velocity. Motor nerve conduction studies and EMG are usually normal.

Although acute sensory neuronopathy bears a superficial resemblance to GBS, distinction can usually be made on clinical grounds and confirmed by electrodiagnostic evaluation. It is likely that most of the sporadic reports of GBS with severe sensory loss constitute examples of sensory neuronopathy.

Acute Pandysautonomia

Autonomic failure of some degree is common in GBS. A syndrome characterized primarily by acute autonomic failure, with minimal sensory and motor
abnormalities, associated with elevated CSF protein, and in which there was
complete spontaneous recovery has also been described.[130–133] In other patients, somatic sensory and motor functions were more involved,[132] sometimes severely,[134] and not all cases recovered. Pathologically, this syndrome is
characterized by some loss of unmyelinated axons with an increased proportion of small diameter unmyelinated axons, suggestive of collateral sprouting. Myelinated axons were largely spared and there is no demyelination or
inflammation. In one patient with severe sensory and autonomic failure there
was severe loss of dorsal root ganglion cells and some loss of neurons from
the peripheral autonomic ganglia.[134] These pathological changes are not
similar to GBS and indicate a primary attack on axons or their cell bodies.
Kinship of this syndrome to GBS rests entirely on the clinical course and
elevated CSF protein and, like the acute sensory neuropathies, it probably is a
distinct entity, rather than a variant of GBS.

Myelopathy

GBS may present in the form of acute paraplegia or quadriplegia, simulating
myelopathy.[135] The presentation may superficially resemble acute myelopathy, especially when there is urinary retention. The confusion may be
compounded when there is significant back pain. With acute myelopathy
from transverse myelitis or spinal cord compression, the leg reflexes may be
absent and occasionally the Babinski reflex is negative. Reflex movement of
the legs, in excess of that which can be volitionally produced, may occasionally be an important clue to the upper motor neuron basis for the
weakness. A clear-cut sensory level on the trunk excludes the diagnosis of
GBS, although some truncal sensory loss may exist from involvement of
segmental spinal nerves. As the illness evolves it becomes much easier to
distinguish myelopathy from GBS, but if there is doubt about the anatomic
localization, an immediate myelogram or magnetic resonance imaging (MRI)
scan may be needed.

Hysteria

Hysterical paralysis is rare and seldom is confused with GBS. Reflexes are
preserved and the neurological signs may have a nonanatomical distribution.
Electrodiagnostic studies of course are normal. More commonly, cases of GBS
are erroneously diagnosed as hysteria early in the evolution of the paralysis.
Paresthesiae may be attributed to hyperventilation and early proximal weakness may result in a disturbance of gait before overt weakness can be detected
by formal strength testing. The confusion may be compounded by preserva-

tion of reflexes early in the disease. Obviously, such confusion may be fatal if a patient should develop autonomic or respiratory problems in an inappropriate setting. In all cases it is better to err on the side of patient safety and admit patients with acute paralysis into an intensive care setting until a certain diagnosis is established.

Summary

The diagnosis of GBS is primarily clinical and is usually not difficult. In developed countries, the occurrence of an acutely evolving, areflexic paralysis, whose onset is heralded by distal paresthesiae, presents little in the way of a diagnostic dilemma. The diagnosis can be confirmed by the characteristic albuminocytologic dissociation in the CSF. Although some variance from the stringent requirements of Guillain are common, significant pleocytosis (>50 cells/mm^3) or normal protein should raise the possibility of an alternative diagnosis or of infection with HIV. Although a host of abnormalities of blood tests has been described, particularly of its antibody profile, none is diagnostically useful. The differential diagnosis includes a wide range of acute paralytic diseases but distinction of GBS from these disorders can almost always be made clinically.

References

1. Guillain G, Barré A, Strohl A. Sur un syndrome de radiculonevrite avec hyperalbuminose du liquide cephalo-rachidien sans reaction cellulaire. Remarques sur les caracters cliniques et graphique des reflexes tendineux. *Bull Soc Med Hop Paris*. 1916;40:1462–1470.
2. Guillain G. Radiculoneuritis with acellular hyperalbuminosis of cerebrospinal fluid. *Arch Neurol Psychiatry*. 1936;36:975–990.
3. Osler LD, Sidell AD. The Guillain-Barré syndrome. The need for exact diagnostic criteria. *N Engl J Med*. 1960;262:964–969.
4. Marshall J. The Landry-Guillain-Barré syndrome. *Brain*. 1963;86:55–66.
5. Wiederholt WC, Mulder DW, Lambert EH. The Landry-Guillain-Barré-Strohl syndrome or polyradiculoneuropathy: historical review, report on 97 patients, and present concepts. *Mayo Clin Proc*. 1964;39:427–451.
6. McFarland HR, Heller GL. Guillain-Barré disease complex: a statement of diagnostic criteria and analysis of 100 cases. *Arch Neurol*. 1966;14:196–201.
7. Ravn H. The Landry-Guillain-Barré syndrome: a survey and a clinical report of 127 cases. *Acta Neurol Scand*. 1967;43(suppl 30):1–64.
8. Masucci EF, Kurtzke JF. Diagnostic criteria for the Guillain-Barré syndrome: an analysis of 50 cases. *J Neurol Sci*. 1971;13:483–501.
9. Loffel NB, Rossi LN, Mumenthaler M, Lutschg J, Ludin H-P. The Landry-Guillain-Barré syndrome. Complications, prognosis and natural history in 123 cases. *J Neurol Sci*. 1977;31:71–79.
10. Asbury AK, Arnason BG, Karp HR, McFarlin DE. Criteria for diagnosis of Guillain-Barré syndrome. *Ann Neurol*. 1978;3:565–566.
11. Asbury AK, Cornblath DR. Assessment of current diagnostic criteria for Guillain-Barré syndrome. *Ann Neurol*. 1990;27(suppl):S21–S24.
12. Queckenstedt H. Uber veranderungen der spinalflussigkeit bei erkrankunger peripherer nerven, insbesondere bei polyneuritis und bei ischias. *Dtsch Ztschr Nervenh*. 1917;57: 316–329.

13. Aring CD. Infectious polyneuritis. *Int Clin.* 1945;4:262–274.
14. Fishman RA. *Cerebrospinal fluid in diseases of the nervous system.* Philadelphia: Saunders; 1980:314–316.
15. McLeod JG, Walsh JC, Prineas JW, Pollard JD. Acute idiopathic polyneuritis. A clinical and electrophysiological follow-up study. *J Neurol Sci.* 1976;27:145–162.
16. Johnson JW. Infectious polyneuritis—diagnostic criteria and military implications. Report of 15 cases. *Med Bull North African Theatre Oper.* 1944;1:149–156.
17. Madigan PS, Marietta SU. Polyradiculoneuritis with report of a case. *Ann Intern Med.* 1938;12:719–726.
18. Debre RL, Theiffrey S. Remarque sur le syndrome de Guillain-Barré chez l'enfants (à propos de 32 observations personelles). *Arch Franc Pediatr.* 1951;8:357–364.
19. Andersson T, Siden A. A clinical study of the Guillain-Barré syndrome. *Acta Neurol Scand.* 1982;66:316–327.
20. Winer JB, Hughes RAC, Osmond C. A prospective study of acute idiopathic neuropathy. I. Clinical features and their prognostic value. *J Neurol Neurosurg Psychiatry.* 1988;51: 605–612.
21. Arnason BGW. Acute inflammatory demyelinating polyradiculoneuropathies. In: Dyck PJ, Thomas PK, Lambert EH, Bunge R, eds. *Peripheral neuropathy.* Philadelphia: Saunders; 1984:2050–2100.
22. Dencker SJ, Swahn B, Ursing B. Protein pattern of the cerebrospinal fluid during the course of acute polyradiculoneuropathy. *Acta Med Scand.* 1964;175:499–506.
23. Link H. Immunoglobulin abnormalities in the Guillain-Barré syndrome. *J Neurol Sci.* 1973; 18:11–23.
24. Link H. Demonstration of oligoclonal immunoglobulin G in Guillain-Barré syndrome. *Acta Neurol Scand.* 1975;52:111–120.
25. Spies JM, Watson JDG, McLeod JG. Guillain-Barré syndrome. A review of 84 cases. *Aust NZ J Med.* 1991;21(suppl 1):183. Abstract.
26. Morley JB, Reynolds EH. Papilloedema and the Landry-Guillain-Barré syndrome. Case reports and a review. *Brain.* 1966;89:205–222.
27. Haymaker W, Kernohan JW. The Landry-Guillain-Barré syndrome. A clinicopathological report of fifty fatal cases and a critique of the literature. *Medicine.* 1949;28:59–141.
28. Fornara P. Contributo allo studio delle meningo-radicoliti. *Clin Pediatr.* 1927;9:403–408.
29. Riser M, Labro P, Planques MJ. De la meningo-neuroniteprimitive aigue avec reaction meningee particulierement intense (hypertrophie troculaire, ataxie, papillite). *Rev Neurol.* 1933;1:1191–1196.
30. Mussio-Fournier JC, Cervino JM, Rocca F, Larossa H, Rufino A. Un cas de meningo-radiculo-nevrite aigue curable, avec xanthochromie et intense lymphocytose dans le liquide cephalo-rachidien, se terminant par une guerison complete. *Rev Neurol.* 1933;2: 104–112.
31. Cornblath DR, McArthur JC, Kennedy PGE, Witte AS, Griffin JW. Inflammatory demyelinating peripheral neuropathies associated with human T-cell lymphotropic virus Type III infection. *Ann Neurol.* 1987;21:32–40.
32. Sterman AB, Nelson S, Barclay P. Demyelinating neuropathy accompanying Lyme disease. *Neurology.* 1982;32:1302–1305.
33. Nyland H, Naess A. Lymphocyte subpopulations in blood and cerebrospinal fluid from patients with acute Guillain-Barré syndrome. *Eur Neurol.* 1978;17:247–252.
34. Nyland H, Naess A. Lymphocytes in peripheral blood from patients with neurological diseases. *Acta Neurol Scand.* 1978;58:272–281.
35. Goust JM, Chenais F, Hames JE, Hames CG, Fudenberg HH, Hogan EL. Abnormal T-cell subpopulations and circulating immune complexes in the Guillain-Barré syndrome and multiple sclerosis. *Neurology.* 1978;28:421–425.
36. Froelich CJ, Searles RP, Davis LE, Goodwin JS. A case of Guillain-Barré syndrome with immunologic abnormalities. *Ann Intern Med.* 1980;93:563–565.
37. Latov N, Gross RB, Kastelman J, et al. Complement-fixing antiperipheral nerve myelin antibodies in patients with inflammatory polyneuritis and with polyneuropathy and paraproteinemia. *Neurology.* 1981;31:1530–1534.
38. Melnick SC. Thirty eight cases of the Guillain-Barré syndrome, an immunologic study. *Br Med J.* 1963;1:368–373.
39. Nyland H, Aarli JA. Guillain-Barré syndrome, demonstration of antibodies to peripheral nerve tissue. *Acta Neurol Scand.* 1978;58:35–43.

40. Lisak RP, Zweiman B, Norman M. Antimyelin antibodies in neurologic disease: IF demonstration. *Arch Neurol*. 1975;32:163–167.
41. Kennedy PGE, Lisak RP. A search for antibodies against glial cells in the serum and cerebrospinal fluid of patients with multiple sclerosis and Guillain-Barré syndrome. *J Neurol Sci*. 1979;44:125–133.
42. Koski CL, Gratz E, Sutherland J, Mayer RF. Clinical correlation with anti-peripheral-nerve myelin antibodies in Guillain-Barré syndrome. *Ann Neurol*. 1986;19:573–577.
43. Ilyas AA, Willison HJ, Quarles RH, et al. Serum antibodies to gangliosides in Guillain-Barré syndrome. *Ann Neurol*. 1988;23:440–447.
44. Ilyas AA, Cook SD, Mithen FA. Anti-GM1 IgA antibodies in Guillain-Barré syndrome. *Peripheral Nerve Study Group Abstracts*. 1991.
45. Latov N, van den Berg LH, Sadio SA, Dhaliwal SK, Sivac M, Walicke PA. Anti-GM1 antibodies in the Guillain-Barré syndrome. *Peripheral Nerve Study Group Abstracts*. 1991.
46. Nobile-Orazio E, Carpo M, Meucci N, Grassi MP, Sciacco M, Scarlato G. Anti-GM1 antibodies in Guillain-Barré syndrome. *Peripheral Nerve Group Abstracts*. 1991.
47. Quarles RH, Ilyas AA, Willison HJ. Antibodies to gangliosides and myelin proteins in Guillain-Barré syndrome. *Ann Neurol*. 1990;27(suppl):S48–S52.
48. Rostami AM, Burns JB, Eccleston PA, Manning MC, Lisak RP, Silberberg DH. Search for antibodies to galactocerebroside in the serum and cerebrospinal fluid in human demyelinating disorders. *Ann Neurol*. 1987;22:381–383.
49. Cook S, Dowling PC, Murray MR, Whitaker JN. Circulating demyelinating factors in acute idiopathic polyneuropathy: myelinotoxic antibody in the Guillain-Barré syndrome. *Arch Neurol*. 1971;24:136–144.
50. Dubois-Dalq M, Buyse M, Buyse G, Gorce F. The action of Guillain-Barré syndrome serum on myelin: a tissue culture and electron microscopic analysis. *J Neurol Sci*. 1971;13:67–83.
51. Feasby TE, Hahn AF, Gilbert JJ. Passive transfer of demyelinating activity in Guillain-Barré polyneuropathy. *Neurology*. 1980;32:1159–1167.
52. Saida T, Saida K, Lisak RP, Brown MJ, Silberberg DH. In vivo demyelinating activity of sera from patients with Guillain-Barré syndrome. *Ann Neurol*. 1982;11:69–75.
53. Sumner AJ, Said G, Idy I, Metral S. Syndrome du Guillain-Barré: effets electrophysiologiques et morphologiques du serum humain introduit dans l'espace endoneural du nerf sciatique du rat. Resultats preliminaires. *Rev Neurol*. 1982;138:17–24.
54. Harrison BM, Hansen LA, Pollard JD, McLeod JG. Demyelination induced by serum from patients with Guillain-Barré syndrome. *Ann Neurol*. 1984;15:163–170.
55. Feit H, Tindall RSA, Glasberg M. Sources of error in the diagnosis of Guillain-Barré syndrome. *Muscle Nerve*. 1982;5:111–117.
56. Morrison EG, Embil JA. Poliomyelitis in North America: the disease is not dead yet. *Can Med Assoc J*. 1987;137:1085–1087.
57. Arlazoroff A, Bleicher Z, Klein C, et al. Vaccine-associated contact poliomyelitis with atypical neurological presentation. *Acta Neurol Scand*. 1987;76:210–214.
58. Floberg JW, Parry GJ, Tahmoush AJ. Poliomyelitis presenting as the Guillain-Barré syndrome. *Muscle Nerve*. 1988;11:961.
59. Querfurth H, Swanson PD. Vaccine-associated paralytic poliomyelitis. Regional case series and review. *Arch Neurol*. 1990;47:541–544.
60. CDSC report. Outbreak of poliomyelitis in Finland. *Br Med J*. 1985;291:41–42.
61. Jubelt B, Lipton HL. Enterovirus infections. In: Vinken PJ, Bruyn GW, Klawans HL, McKendall PR, eds. *Handbook of clinical neurology*. Amsterdam: Elsevier/North Holland Biomedical Press; 1989; 12(56):307–347.
62. Gibbons A. New "China syndrome" puzzle. *Science*. 1991;251:26.
63. McKhann GM, Cornblath DR, Ho T, et al. Acute paralytic disease of children and young adults in Northern China. *Ann Neurol*. 1991;30:260. Abstract.
64. Cornblath DR, McKhann GM, Ho T, et al. Electrophysiology of acute paralytic disease of children and young adults in Northern China. *Ann Neurol*. 1991;30:260. Abstract.
65. Ramos-Alvarez M, Bessudo L, Sabin AB. Paralytic syndromes associated with non-inflammatory cytoplasmic or nuclear neuronopathy. Acute paralytic disease in Mexican children neuropathologically distinguishable from Landry-Guillain-Barré syndrome. *JAMA*. 1969;207:1481–1492.
66. Tucker T, Layzer RL. Subacute reversible motor neuron disease. *Neurology*. 1985;35(suppl 1): 108. Abstract.

67. Jackson CE, Woodard C, Barohn RJ. Acute motor neuronopathy simulating Guillain-Barré syndrome. *Neurology*. 1991;41:133. Abstract.
68. Horstman DM. Epidemiology of poliomyelitis and allied diseases. *Yale J Biol Med*. 1963;36:5–12.
69. Plum F. Sensory loss with poliomyelitis. *Neurology*. 1956;6:166–167.
70. McDowell FH, Plum F. Arterial hypertension associated with acute anterior poliomyelitis. *N Engl J Med*. 1951;245:241–244.
71. Baker AB, Matzke HA, Brown JR. Poliomyelitis VI. The hypothalamus. *Arch Neurol Psychiatry*. 1952;68:16–21.
72. Kinnunen E, Farkkila M, Hovi T, Juntunen J, Weckstrom P. Incidence of Guillain-Barré syndrome during a nationwide oral poliovirus vaccine campaign. *Neurology*. 1989;39:1034–1036.
73. Abbott KH. Tick paralysis: a review. *Mayo Clin Proc*. 1943;18:39–45, 59–62.
74. Stanbury JB, Huyck JH. Tick paralysis: a critical review. *Medicine*. 1945;24:219–242.
75. Rodichok LD, Barron KD. Neurologic complications of bee sting, tick bite, and scorpion bite. In: Vinken PJ, Bruyn GW, eds. *Handbook of clinical neurology*. Amsterdam: Elsevier-North Holland Biomedical Press; 1979;37:107–114.
76. Kaire GH. Isolation of tick paralysis toxin from Ixodes holocyclus. *Toxicon*. 1966;4:91–97.
77. Kocan AA. Tick paralysis. *J Am Vet Med Assoc*. 1988;192:1498–1500.
78. Wright SW, Trott AT. North American tick-borne diseases. *Ann Emerg Med*. 1988;17:964–972.
79. Cherington M, Snyder R. Tick paralysis, neurophysiologic studies. *N Engl J Med*. 1968;278:95–97.
80. Swift TR, Ignacio OJ. Tick paralysis: electrophysiologic studies. *Neurology*. 1975;25:1130–1133.
81. Murnaghan M. Conduction block of terminal somatic motor fibers in tick paralysis. *Can J Biochem Physiol*. 1960;38:287–295.
82. Emmons O, McLennan H. Failure of acetylcholine release in tick paralysis. *Nature*. 1959;183:465–467.
83. McLennan H, Oikawa I. Changes in function of the neuromuscular junction occurring in tick paralysis. *Can J Physiol Pharmacol*. 1972;50:53–58.
84. Gauci M, Stone BF, Thong YH. Detection in allergic individuals of IgE specific for the Australian paralysis tick, Ixodes holocyclus. *Int Arch Allergy Appl Immun*. 1988;85:190–193.
85. Scheid W. Diphtherial paralysis. An analysis of 2292 cases of diphtheria in adults, which included 174 cases of polyneuritis. *J Nerv Ment Dis*. 1952;116:1095–1101.
86. Paley RG, Truelove SC. Diphtheria in the army in the United Kingdom. A study of its complications. *J Roy Army Med Corps*. 1948;90:109–116.
87. Walshe FMR. On the pathogenesis of diphtheritic paralysis. *Q J Med*. 1918;11:191–204.
88. Brown MR. The mechanism involved in polyneuritis as exemplified by post-diphtheritic polyneuritis. *Ann Intern Med*. 1952;36:786–791.
89. McDonald WI, Kocen RS. Diphtheritic neuropathy. In: Dyck PJ, Thomas PK, Lambert EH, Bunge R, eds. *Peripheral Neuropathy*. Philadelphia: Saunders; 1984:2010–2017.
90. Fisher CM, Adams RD. Diphtheritic polyneuritis—a pathological study. *J Neuropathol Exp Neurol*. 1956;15:243–268.
91. Kurdi A, Abdul-Kader M. Clinical and electrophysiological studies of diphtheritic neuritis in Jordan. *J Neurol Sci*. 1979;42:243–250.
92. Mills AR, Passmore R. Pelagic paralysis. *Lancet*. 1988;1:161–164.
93. Sakamoto Y, Lockey RF, Krzanowski JJ. Shellfish and fish poisoning related to toxic dinoflagellates. *South Med J*. 1987;80:866–872.
94. Canedo J, Sanders DB. Peripheral electrophysiological studies in ciguatera. *Neurology*. 1988;383:308. Abstract.
95. Ayyar DR, Mullaly WJ. Ciguatera: clinical and electrophysiological observations. *Neurology*. 28:354. Abstract.
96. Weller RO, Mitchell J, Daves GD, Jr. Buckthorn (Karwinskia humboldtiana) Toxins. In: Spencer PS, Schaumburg HH, eds. *Experimental and clinical neurotoxicology*. Baltimore: Williams and Wilkins; 1980:336–347.
97. Padron-Puyou F. Estudio clinico-experimental de la paralisis por Karwinskia humboldtiana ("tullidora") en niños. *Gac Med Mexico*. 1951;81:299–312.
98. Sorensen AWS, With TK. Persistent paresis after porphyric attacks. *South Afr Med J*. 1971;45(special issue):101–103.

99. Albers JW. *Porphyric neuropathy*. In: *Handbook of Peripheral Neuropathies*. Mendell JR, Griffin JW, Cornblath DR, eds. New York; Marcel Dekker (in press).
100. Ridley A. Porphyric neuropathy. In: Dyck PJ, Thomas PK, Lambert EH, Bunge R, eds. *Peripheral Neuropathy*. Philadelphia: Saunders; 1984:1704–1716.
101. Albers JW, Robertson WC, Daube JR. Electrodiagnostic findings in acute porphyric neuropathy. *Muscle Nerve*. 1978;1:292–296.
102. Carlson SE, Rhee S, Blaivas M, Feldman EL, Albers JW. Variegate porphyria presenting as an acute demyelinating neuropathy. *Muscle Nerve*. 1988;11:960. Abstract.
103. Moore PM, Fauci AS. Neurological manifestations of systemic vasculitis. A retrospective and prospective study of the clinicopathologic features and responses to therapy in 25 patients. *Am J Med*. 1981;71:517–524.
104. Parry GJG. Mononeuropathy multiplex. (AAEE case report #11). *Muscle Nerve*. 1985;8: 493–498.
105. Kissell JT, Slivka AP, Warmolts JR, Mendell JR. The clinical spectrum of necrotizing angiopathy of the peripheral nervous system. *Ann Neurol*. 1985;18:251–257.
106. Moore PM, Cupps TR. Neurological complications of vasculitis. *Ann Neurol*. 1983;14:155–167.
107. Jamieson PW, Giuliani MJ, Martinez AJ. Necrotizing angiopathy presenting with multifocal conduction blocks. *Neurology*. 1991;41:442–444.
108. Wees SJ, Sunwoo IN, Oh SJ. Sural nerve biopsy in systemic necrotizing vasculitis. *Am J Med*. 1981;71:525–532.
109. Carrol WM, Mastaglia FL. "Locked-in coma" in post-infective polyneuropathy. *Arch Neurol*. 1979;36:46–47.
110. Loeb C, Mancardi GL, Tabaton M. Locked-in syndrome in acute inflammatory poly-radiculoneuropathy. *Eur Neurol*. 1984;23:137–140.
111. Gherardi RK, Chariot P, Vanderstigel M, et al. Organic arsenic-induced Guillain-Barré-like syndrome due to melarsoprol: a clinical, electrophysiological and pathological study. *Muscle Nerve*. 1990;13:637–645.
112. Donofrio PD, Wilbourn AJ, Albers JW, Rogers L, Salanga V, Greenberg HS. Acute arsenic intoxication presenting as Guillain-Barré-like syndrome. *Muscle Nerve*. 1987;10:114–120.
113. Schlumpf U, Meyer M, Ulrich J, Friede RL. Neurologic complications induced by gold treatment. *Arthritis Rheum*. 1983;26:825–831.
114. Katrak SM, Pollock M, O'Brien CP, et al. Clinical and morphological features of gold neuropathy. *Brain*. 1980;103:671–693.
115. Dick DJ, Raman D. The Guillain-Barré syndrome following gold therapy. *Scand J Rheumatol*. 1982;11:119–120.
116. Roquer J, Herraiz J, Maymo J, Olive A, Carbonell J. Miller-Fisher syndrome (Guillain-Barré syndrome with ophthalmoplegia) during treatment of gold salts in a patient with rheuma-toid arthritis. *Arthritis Rheum*. 1985;28:838–839.
117. Vernay D, Dubost JJ, Thevant JP, Sauvezie B, Rampon S. "Choree fibrillaire de Morvan" followed by Guillain-Barré syndrome in a patient receiving gold therapy. *Arthritis Rheum*. 1986;29:1413–1414.
118. Namba T, Nolte CT, Jackrel J, Grob D. Poisoning due to organophosphate insecticides. Acute and chronic manifestations. *Am J Med*. 1971;50:475–492.
119. Wadia RS, Sadagopan C, Amin RB, Sardesai HV. Neurological manifestations of organo-phosphorus insecticide poisoning. *J Neurol Neurosurg Psychiatry*. 1974;37:841–847.
120. Estrin WJ, Parry GJ. Neurotoxicology. In: La Dou J, ed. *Occupational medicine*. Norwalk: Appleton & Lange; 1990:267–274.
121. Fisher JR. Guillain-Barré syndrome following organophosphate poisoning. *JAMA*. 1977; 238:1950–1951.
122. Walsh JC, McLeod JG. Alcoholic neuropathy: an electrophysiological and histological study. *J Neurol Sci*. 1970;10:457–469.
123. Tabaraud F, Vallat JM, Hugon J, Ramiandrisoa H, Dumas M, Signoret JL. Acute or subacute alcoholic neuropathy mimicking Guillain-Barré syndrome. *J Neurol Sci*. 1990;97:195–205.
124. Watson JDG, Spies JM, McLeod JG. Chronic inflammatory demyelinating polyneuropathy-neuropathy. A review of 74 patients. *Aust NZ J Med*. 1991;21(suppl 1):178. Abstract.
125. Sterman AB, Schaumburg HH, Asbury AK. The acute sensory neuronopathy syndrome: a distinct clinical entity. *Ann Neurol*. 1980;7:354–358.
126. Windebank AJ, Blexrud MD, Dyck PJ, Daube JR, Karnes JL. The syndrome of acute sensory neuropathy: clinical features and electrophysiological and pathological changes. *Neurology*. 1990;40:584–591.

127. Horwich MS, Cho L, Porro RS, Posner JB. Subacute sensory neuropathy: a remote effect of carcinoma. *Ann Neurol*. 1977;2:7–19.
128. Malinow K, Yannakakis GD, Glusman SM, et al. Subacute sensory neuronopathy secondary to dorsal root ganglionitis in primary Sjogren's syndrome. *Ann Neurol*. 1986;20:535–537.
129. Parry GJ, Bredesen DE. Sensory neuropathy with low-dose pyridoxine. *Neurology*. 1985;35:1466–1468.
130. Thomashefsky AF, Horwitz SF, Feingold MH. Acute autonomic neuropathy. *Neurology*. 1972;22:251–255.
131. Young RR, Asbury AK, Corbett JL, Adams RD. Pure pandysautonomia with recovery. Description and discussion of diagnostic criteria. *Brain*. 1975;98:613–636.
132. Appenzeller O, Kornfeld M. Acute pandysautonomia. *Arch Neurol*. 1973;29:334–339.
133. Hart RG, Kanter MC. Acute autonomic neuropathy. Two cases and a clinical review. *Arch Intern Med*. 1990;150:2373–2376.
134. Fagius J, Westerberg C-E, Olsson Y. Acute pandysautonomia and severe sensory deficit with poor recovery. A clinical, neurophysiological and pathological case study. *J Neurol Neurosurg Psychiatry*. 1983;46:725–733.
135. Passmore AP, Taylor IC, McConnell JG. Acute Guillain-Barré syndrome presenting as acute spinal cord compression in an elderly woman. *J Roy Soc Med*. 1990;83:333–334.

4

Electrodiagnostic Evaluation

The early and accurate diagnosis of Guillain-Barré syndrome (GBS) depends primarily on nerve conduction studies. They also provide important prognostic information, especially when combined with needle electromyography. Carefully performed nerve conduction studies of multiple nerves, including cranial nerves and proximal segments of spinal nerves if indicated, are almost always abnormal even when the cerebrospinal fluid (CSF) protein is normal. Furthermore, abnormalities of nerve conduction are more diagnostically specific and, despite the associated discomfort, studies can usually be repeated more frequently and with better patient acceptance than repeated lumbar puncture. In addition to standard motor and sensory nerve conduction studies, useful information can sometimes be obtained from studies of late responses (F-waves and H-reflexes), blink reflexes, and somatosensory evoked potentials. The recently developed technique of electromagnetic nerve stimulation is still limited by technical considerations but, in the future, may offer distinct advantages in evaluating proximal nerve segments. The electrophysiological diagnosis of GBS requires the demonstration of the characteristic changes associated with acute demyelination. These changes have been established as the physiological correlates of demyelination by numerous investigators.[1-6]

Morphological Basis for Nerve Conduction Abnormalities

GBS is an acute, multifocal, demyelinating neuropathy that evolves over days to weeks. The initial pathological lesion of myelinated axons is macrophage-mediated demyelination, followed by Schwann cell proliferation and re-myelination. In addition, there is variable axonal degeneration, which is occasionally severe and may rarely be the predominant pathological finding. The earliest lesions are found in the most proximal and most distal portions of motor axons; that is, in ventral roots and terminal, intramuscular aboriza-tions. Later, demyelination is found along the length of many nerve trunks. The nature and distribution of the pathological lesions and the pattern of evolution gives rise to scattered lesions, throughout the peripheral nervous system, at different stages of demyelination and remyelination and with different degrees of associated axonal degeneration.

The principle electrophysiological correlates of these morphological changes are conduction block, conduction slowing, and differential temporal dispersion of compound action potentials, the compound muscle action potential (CMAP) in particular. To understand the clinical electrodiagnostic findings at the different stages of evolution of GBS requires an understanding of the pathophysiological changes that accompany the morphological changes described.

Conduction Block

DEFINITION OF CONDUCTION BLOCK IN ACUTE NEUROPATHY

The definition of conduction block has generated a great deal of recent controversy, at least in chronic neuropathies. However, in acute GBS, there should be no difficulty in recognizing conduction block, even of mild degree. There is normally only a small drop in the amplitude of the CMAP when responses from proximal and distal stimulus sites are compared. This fall in amplitude is due to the slight temporal dispersion of the CMAP, resulting from separation of slower from faster conducting electrical impulses, which occurs over a long nerve segment. In normal humans, this amplitude drop should not exceed 15% to 20% in the arm nerves, between wrist and elbow.[6-11] In acute situations, an amplitude drop of more than 20% is abnormal and more than 30% almost certainly indicates conduction block, provided that there is no temporal dispersion. However, when a demyelinating neuropathy has progressed for more than a few days, the range of conduction velocities in the motor axons increases dramatically and temporal dispersion develops. Temporal dispersion of the CMAP results in an amplitude drop, accom-panied by an increase in the negative peak duration. Therefore, amplitude reduction alone is insufficient to define conduction block unless the negative peak duration increases by less than 15%. In acute neuropathies, these negative peak amplitude and duration criteria are probably sufficient to establish conduction block. Unfortunately, these same criteria have been uncritically applied to chronic situations, which has resulted in identifica-tion of "conduction block" in a host of chronic diseases, a problem that is discussed below.

CONDUCTION BLOCK IN ACUTE EXPERIMENTAL DEMYELINATION

The principle electrophysiological abnormality that results from acute de-myelination is conduction block, which is best demonstrated in motor axons. In phenomenological terms, this indicates that axons are incapable of trans-mitting electrical impulses over a focal (demyelinated) nerve segment but can conduct normally both proximal and distal to that segment. With complete focal conduction block, without accompanying axonal degeneration, a nor-mal motor response can be elicited by stimulation distal to the lesion but no response can be elicited with proximal stimulation. With partial conduction block, the proximally elicited response is still present but is of reduced amplitude. This can best be demonstrated in experimental animals by inject-ing demyelinating antisera, or some other demyelinating agent, into the sciatic nerve.[12,13] When antibodies to galactocerebroside, a component of myelin, are injected into the sciatic nerve of a rat there is rapidly evolving, focal conduction block confined to the site of injection (Fig. 4–1). That is, the

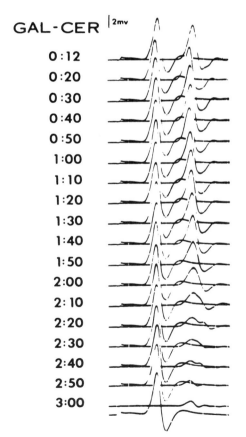

GAL-CER $|^{2mv}$

0:12
0:20
0:30
0:40
0:50
1:00
1:10
1:20
1:30
1:40
1:50
2:00
2:10
2:20
2:30
2:40
2:50
3:00

Figure 4–1. This series of traces shows the evolution of almost com-plete conduction block in the sciatic nerve of a rat that has been injected intraneurally with demyelinating anti-serum (GAL-CER). The compound muscle action potential elicited with distal stimulation, on the left, does not change during the 3 hr after anti-serum injection. The amplitude of the proximal response falls rapidly to reach a nadir about 3 hr after injec-tion, indicating severe conduction block in the motor fibers, but there is no conduction slowing. These results indicate that the essential feature of acute demyelination is conduction block, not conduction slowing. (From ref. 13, with permission.)

CMAP amplitude elicited by stimulation of the nerve distally, at the ankle, remains unchanged while the amplitude of the response elicited by stimulation proximally, at the sciatic notch, rapidly falls and eventually reaches a nadir about 3 hr after antiserum injection. With this acute experimental lesion, in which there is demyelination but no remyelination or axonal degeneration, it is possible to examine the electrophysiological consequences of pure demyelination. First, the distal response remains entirely normal. Second, the amplitude of the proximal response progressively falls but there is no temporal dispersion of the CMAP. Finally, there is little or no slowing of maximal conduction velocity, at least when measured using techniques analogous to the conventional techniques used to measure motor nerve conduction velocity in humans. Experimental demyelination can also be produced by application of a tiny drop of antiserum to the ventral root.[14] Conduction can then be studied over very short segments, covering only a few internodes, in single myelinated axons, and the events occurring at individual nodes of Ranvier can be evaluated. Using this technique it has been shown that before the development of conduction block, there is a profound delay in nodal depolarization producing severe slowing of conduction velocity when it is measured over these very short distances. The effect of this nodal delay confined to a few nodes is diluted by normal conduction over the rest of the nerve so that, with very localized demyelination, conduction slowing is not seen using conventional techniques. As demyelination becomes more widespread and the delay in nodal depolarization is repeated simultaneously at multiple internodes along the length of the nerve, conduction slowing may be seen; even when this does occur propagation of longitudinal current becomes insecure and conduction block is a more likely result. Thus, the *sine qua non* of acute demyelination is conduction block, not conduction slowing.

CONDUCTION BLOCK IN EARLY GBS

A clinical situation analogous to experimental, antiserum-induced, acute demyelination occurs during the earliest stages of GBS, when peripheral nerves are undergoing acute demyelination, with little, if any, remyelination. At this time, the only abnormality of nerve conduction may be conduction block without slowing. However, to make a confident diagnosis of conduction block it is necessary to stimulate the nerve on both sides of a focal demyelinative lesion. Since the earliest lesions in GBS are most often found in ventral roots and distal intramuscular nerve branches, stimulation both proximal and distal to the lesion is not possible and conduction block can only be implied. For ventral root lesions, conduction block is often implied from the absence or impersistence of F-waves[15,16] (Fig. 4–2). However, absent F-waves may occasionally be found in normal individuals so that in a given patient the absence of F-waves cannot be construed as indicating definite proximal conduction block. Nonetheless, the absence of F-waves in a patient with acutely evolving paralysis and especially in young people in whom F-waves are more easily elicited does provide strong support for the diagnosis

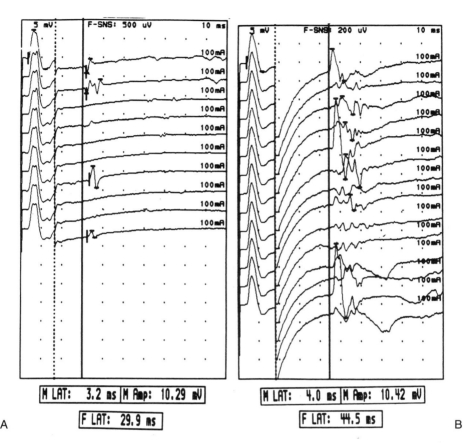

Figure 4–2. The evolution of changes in ulnar nerve F-waves during the first 4 weeks after the onset of mild GBS. The initial study (**A**) was performed 4 days after the onset of symptoms when there was mild weakness in the hands. The distal motor latency (*M LAT*), CMAP amplitude (*M Amp*), F-wave latency (*F LAT*), and conduction velocity between axilla and wrist (not shown) are all normal but there is impersistence of F-wave firing, suggesting partial conduction block, proximal to the axilla. At the time of the second study (**B**), performed 3 weeks later, M LAT has increased but M Amp and conduction velocity remain normal. There is severe prolongation of F LAT and chronodispersion of F-waves but they are now fully persistent, indicating reversal of proximal, conduction block and development of conduction slowing accompanying remyelination.

of GBS. Similarly, for the most distal lesions, occurring in the terminal, intramuscular arborization of the motor axon, pure conduction block would produce only a fall in the amplitude of the distal CMAP, with little prolongation of distal motor latency. Thus, the earliest electrodiagnostic abnormalities seen in GBS may be absent or impersistent F-waves and a low amplitude CMAP. Since these findings may be seen in normal individuals, or in other neuropathies, the nerve conduction studies in GBS may be nondiagnostic if performed during the first few days after the onset of neurological symptoms and studies need to be repeated.

As the disease progresses, demyelination is more likely to occur along the intermediate portion of nerve trunks, resulting in conduction block, which is easy to demonstrate because the nerve can be stimulated on either side of the demyelinating lesion (Fig. 4–3). However, by the time conduction block can be demonstrated at these sites there may be widespread, patchy involvement of all levels of the peripheral nerves, with conduction slowing and temporal dispersion as well as conduction block.

CONDUCTION BLOCK IN CHRONIC NEUROPATHIES

As previously mentioned, there is normally only a small drop in CMAP amplitude between distal and proximal stimulus sites (Fig. 4–4). Reductions in amplitude of 15% to 40% have been suggested as minimal criteria for the diagnosis of conduction block[6,8–10,17] based on experience with acute demyelinating neuropathies. When the range of conduction velocities in a nerve is increased by demyelination or when there is chronic axon loss with reinnervation of muscle by collateral sprouting of remaining motor axons, as occurs in chronic neuropathies and motor neuron disease, amplitude and area changes are common and may be erroneously attributed to conduction block. For example, with chronic demyelination there is an increased range of conduction velocities with temporal dispersion and reduced amplitude of a

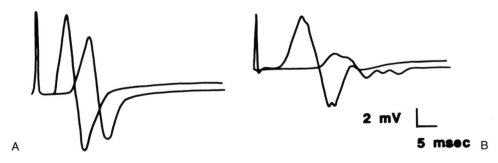

A   2 mV

5 msec B

Figure 4–3. The evolution of acute conduction block in a 33-year-old woman with distal paresthesiae and moderately severe global weakness. The first median motor nerve conduction study (**A**) was performed 3 days after the onset of symptoms. The distal CMAP amplitude, distal motor latency, and forearm conduction velocity are all normal. However, there is a 30% fall in CMAP amplitude between wrist and elbow with minimal temporal dispersion, suggesting acute conduction block. Very few F-waves could be elicited (15%), suggesting proximal conduction block, but those present were of normal latency. The significance of these early conduction changes becomes fully evident in the follow-up study (**B**) performed 8 days later. The distal CMAP amplitude has fallen from 8.6 to 5.7 mV and the response is mildly dispersed. There is now a 70% fall in CMAP amplitude between wrist and elbow with marked temporal dispersion of the proximal response. The distal motor latency has increased from 4.4 to 6.0 ms and forearm conduction velocity has fallen from 50.0 to 33.0 m/s. F-waves were more frequent (72%) but responses were chronodispersed and the minimum latency was markedly prolonged (46 ms). The second study shows a combination of conduction block, conduction slowing, and temporal dispersion.

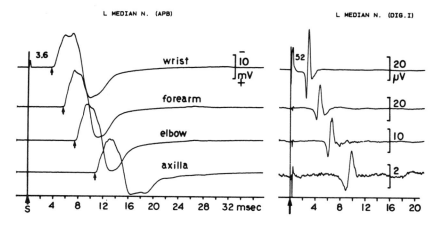

Figure 4–4. Median motor and sensory nerve conduction in a normal individual. The CMAP amplitude shows a negligible decline in amplitude as the nerve is stimulated progressively more proximally. In contrast, there is a dramatic fall in the SNAP amplitude recorded at the sites of stimulation for the motor study. (Modified from ref. 20, with permission.)

proximally elicited response. The increased negative peak duration of the dispersed proximal CMAP distinguishes this type of amplitude change from conduction block. However, significant reductions in amplitude without a significant increase in negative peak duration may occur due to interphase cancellation. A CMAP comprises the summated electrical potentials of its component parts (the motor units). When there is a narrow range of conduction velocities and the electrical impulse traverses only a short distance, the motor units, which make up the CMAP, fire in a highly synchronous fashion and there is little opportunity for cancellation of the negative phase of one motor unit potential by the positive phase of another. As the electrical volley traverses longer and longer nerve segments, there is progressive desynchronization of the electrical volley until some interphase cancellation is inevitable and results in loss of amplitude of the CMAP, out of proportion to the increased duration of the negative peak.[18] In normal motor nerves there is negligible amplitude reduction as a result of interphase cancellation because the long duration of individual motor unit potentials (5–15 ms) necessitates a large phase shift before significant phase interactions occur (Fig. 4–4). Furthermore, when there is equal slowing of conduction in all motor fibers, as usually occurs in the hereditary demyelinating neuropathies, the range of conduction velocities may not be much altered so that amplitude changes due to interphase cancellation may be minimal despite severe slowing. However, when there is an increased range of conduction velocities, as occurs in acquired demyelinating neuropathies, major phase shifts can occur and there is a reduction in the amplitude of the CMAP that is out of proportion to the increased negative peak duration. This may be mistaken for conduction block but is due to interphase cancellation. Phase cancellation may also occur when there is chronic denervation even in the absence of demyelination, as occurs in chronic axonal neuropathies or motor neuron disease. When motor units are lost, terminal collateral sprouting of surviving units produces increased polyphasia of the motor unit potentials with an increased likelihood of phase interaction and cancellation.[19] In addition, there are fewer motor units and phase cancellation in a small number of giant, polyphasic motor unit potentials may have an inordinately large effect on the amplitude of the surface-recorded CMAP. As a result, patients with chronic axon loss from any cause may have significant reductions in amplitude as progressively longer nerve segments are studied, and this may be misinterpreted as conduction block. Rhee et al.[18] used computer simulation to show that interphase cancellation can account for at least a 50% reduction in amplitude due to interphase cancellation associated with loss of motor units. However, amplitude changes occur smoothly along the nerve as progressively more distant sites are stimulated (Fig. 4–5). By contrast, amplitude and wave form changes associated with focal demyelination, whether they are due to conduction block or temporal dispersion and interphase cancellation, are confined to restricted segments of nerve. From the diagnostic point of view, changes in amplitude, wave form, and conduction velocity that are restricted to focal nerve segments have essentially the same implication; that is, they indicate focal demyelination. However, there are important functional differences: conduction block causes loss of function whereas focal slowing and dispersion has no significant functional consequences.

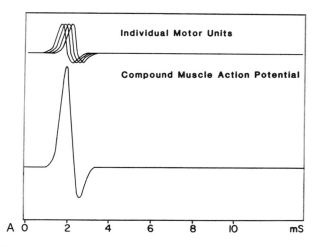

Figure 4–5. The simulated effect of progressive dispersion of individual motor units on the compound muscle action potential amplitude and wave form. When there is almost synchronous firing of motor units (**A**), they summate to form a large amplitude CMAP with a compact, biphasic wave form. (Figure continued on next page)

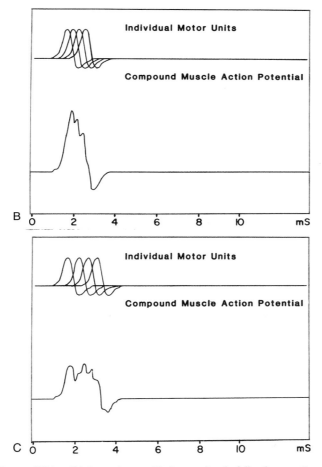

Figure 4–5, Cont. With mild desynchrony (**B**) the amplitude falls, the negative peak duration increases, and the wave form becomes multiphasic. As the desynchronization increases (**C**), the changes in amplitude and wave form become more severe. This sequence is representative of the gradual change in amplitude and wave form that occurs as progressively longer segments of nerve are studied in patients with an increased range of conduction velocities but no conduction block.

Phase cancellation produces major amplitude changes in nerve action potentials, such as the sensory nerve action potentials recorded during routine nerve conduction studies, even in normal nerves. The compound nerve action potential is made up of the summated spike potentials of individual large myelinated axons in the nerve. These have a duration of 1 ms or less and, as a result, a much smaller phase shift results in the interaction of the positive phase of one spike and the negative phase of another. Therefore, the minimal dispersion that occurs in normal nerves may produce significant interphase cancellation. The amplitude of a compound nerve action potential therefore depends on the length of nerve over which conduction is measured. It is normal for the amplitude of the sensory nerve action potential, recorded in the median or ulnar nerve at the elbow, to fall to 30% to 50% of the amplitude recorded at the wrist[20] (Fig. 4–4). When the range of conduction velocities in a sensory nerve is increased by demyelination, this results in a severe reduction of the sensory nerve action potential amplitude, even when there is no conduction block. Dispersion of the response can be seen only with computer averaging of many evoked responses.

Phase cancellation in giant motor units in partially denervated muscles almost certainly accounts for the observation that patients with classical amyotrophic lateral sclerosis may have "conduction block."[21] If there is an alteration of amplitude between distal and proximal sites of stimulation this should be interpreted only as "suggestive of conduction block."[22] Further electrophysiological investigation can then be undertaken to determine whether there is true conduction block. First, it should be demonstrated that the amplitude change occurs abruptly over a short nerve segment, rather than gradually, along the length of the nerve. This can be achieved by incremental short-segment stimulation, either percutaneously or using a monopolar needle as the stimulating cathode. Second, with an intramuscular coaxial needle as the recording electrode, it may be possible to record motor units that are present with distal but not proximal stimulation, or motor units that can be elicited by distal stimulation cannot be volitionally activated. Third, the waveform of the electrically evoked CMAP should resemble the summated individual, surface-recorded motor unit potentials (MUPs) elicited by maximal volitional contraction. In a cooperative patient, there is conduction block if the electrically elicited CMAP cannot be resynthesized from the surface-recorded unitary volitional responses. If these criteria cannot be met, amplitude/area changes should be interpreted with caution.

Conduction Slowing and Temporal Dispersion

As already discussed, acute, focal, experimental demyelination does not produce conduction slowing when measured using conventional techniques despite profound delays at individual affected nodes of Ranvier. However, if focal demyelinating lesions are widely scattered along the length of a nerve fiber, the individual nodal delays may summate sufficiently to produce marked conduction slowing, even using conventional techniques. In GBS, if the demyelinating lesions are widely distributed, marked conduction slowing can be seen during the acute stage of the disease. Thus, when demyelination is concentrated proximally, the latency of any F-waves that can be recorded may be prolonged; there may also be marked chronodispersion of F-waves with some having normal latencies and others having prolonged latencies. Similarly, when the most distal motor nerve segments are involved, the distal motor latency may be prolonged, even early in the course of the disease, if enough nodes are affected by the demyelination. The distal motor latency may also be more obviously affected because the much shorter distances over which it is measured make it less likely that the effect of localized slowing will be diluted by normal conduction velocity over the remainder of the nerve segment being evaluated. Nonetheless, such widespread demyelination so reduces the safety factor for electrical impulse propagation that it is more likely to produce block.

MECHANISMS OF CONDUCTION SLOWING AND TEMPORAL DISPERSION

Conduction velocity along an axon is determined entirely by the delay that occurs at each node of Ranvier.[1,23] Conduction along an internode depends solely on the cable properties of the axon and is extremely rapid, resulting in negligible internodal delay.[14,23] Therefore, conduction velocity is determined by the delay at each node and the number of nodes. In acute demyelination there is no change in the number of nodes but there is a marked increased in the delay at each affected node in which conduction is not completely blocked. This delay results primarily from the additional time taken to overcome the increased nodal capacitance associated with the demyelination. Increased nodal delay can be measured at every affected node and, if repeated at enough nodes, conduction slowing can be measured.

As an axon remyelinates, a number of factors conspire to produce conduction slowing. First, there is an increase in the number of nodes of Ranvier. When a demyelinated nerve remyelinates, the territory of the axon invested by myelin derived originally from a single Schwann cell is remyelinated by several new Schwann cells, with a proportional increase in the number of nodes. Second, at the time conduction is reestablished, each new node is very rudimentary, with a greater area of nodal axolemma exposed to the extracellular fluid (ECF) and therefore greater nodal capacitance and an increased delay at each node. Finally, each new internode is invested with fewer myelin lamellae so that there is increased internodal axial current leakage and less longitudinal current arrives at the node, compounding the delay at individual nodes. As myelin thickness increases and the nodal architecture matures, conduction velocity increases, but the original conduction velocity may never be completely restored. When conduction velocity is measured in nerve populations, the variable degree of demyelination and remyelination in individual axons increases the range of conduction velocities, resulting in temporal dispersion of the compound action potential.

Conduction Slowing and Temporal Dispersion in Experimental Demyelination

If experimental animals with complete, focal conduction block are sequentially studied after antiserum injection, the response elicited by distal stimulation remains unchanged but, after a delay of about a week, a small response

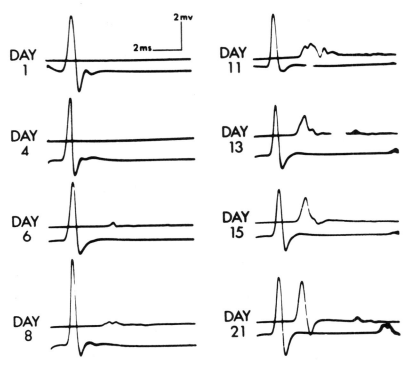

Figure 4–6. These traces show recovery from complete conduction block after intraneural injection of demyelinating antiserum. A small proximal response with very slow conduction velocity is first seen on day 6. As recovery occurs the latency of the proximal response shortens as maximal conduction velocity increases. In addition, the proximal response first becomes dispersed and then progressively more synchronous as the range of conduction velocities reduces. There is no significant change in the distal response. (From ref. 13, with permission.)

appears with stimulation proximal to the site of injection[13] (Fig. 4–6). The initial response has an extremely long latency and conduction velocity across the restricted region of demyelination has been estimated to be as low as 2 m/s at the time conduction is first reestablished. Once the first proximal electrical response is seen there is rapid return of normal clinical function, at least insofar as it can be evaluated in rats. However, the electrophysiological studies remain markedly abnormal. There is slowing of maximal conduction velocity and temporal dispersion of the proximal response. Morphologically, the return of the first proximally elicited response coincides with the onset of remyelination, with from two to eight myelin lamellae being required to reestablish conduction.[24] As more axons remyelinate, the CMAP becomes more synchronous and amplitude increases, but it remains dispersed because of differential slowing in axons at different stages of remyelination, producing an increased range of conduction velocities. Thus, the electrophysiological correlate of remyelination is marked slowing of maximal conduction velocity with dispersion of the CMAP across the site of demyelination. In these experimental animals, as remyelination progresses, maximal conduction velocity increases and the CMAP becomes progressively less dispersed; by 5 to 6 weeks it has returned completely to normal.

CONDUCTION SLOWING AND TEMPORAL DISPERSION IN GBS

In patients with GBS, as the disease evolves, slowing becomes more prominent and differential temporal dispersion develops (Fig. 4–7). These changes parallel the appearance of more widespread foci of demyelination as well as the onset of remyelination. This pattern of marked conduction slowing and temporal dispersion is perhaps the most characteristic clinical electrodiagnostic feature of the disease. As remyelination occurs in the nerve roots, F-waves reappear, with marked latency prolongation and chronodispersion of responses. As remyelination occurs in distal, intramuscular nerves, the CMAP elicited by distal stimulation becomes markedly dispersed and distal motor latency becomes even more prolonged. As remyelination occurs along the length of nerve trunks, temporal dispersion increases between adjacent sites of stimulation. Thus, patients with GBS usually show various combinations of conduction block, differential dispersion, and conduction slowing

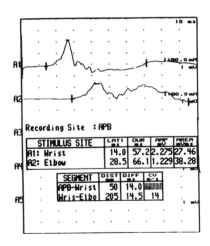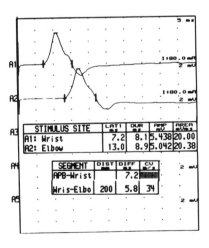

Figure 4–7. Motor nerve conduction in the median nerve from elbow to wrist, performed 6 weeks (**left**) and 6 months (**right**) after the onset of severe GBS. At 6 weeks, when recovery of strength was already occurring, there is severe latency prolongation (14.0 ms) and dispersion of the distal response (*upper trace*). The proximal response (*lower trace*) is even more dispersed so that the amplitude has dropped by almost 50%. Maximal conduction velocity is severely slowed (14 m/s) between elbow and wrist. At 6 months strength had returned to normal and conduction had improved but remained severely abnormal. The distal motor latency has reduced to 7.2 ms and conduction velocity has increased to 34 m/s. There is now only mild dispersion of the responses and no differential dispersion between elbow and wrist, indicating that the range of conduction velocities has considerably narrowed. (Figure provided courtesy of Dr. Jean Teasley.)

involving proximal, distal, and intermediate segments of nerves, depending on the time of the study in relationship to the onset of neurological symptoms. With time, there is a progressive increase in the conduction velocity and the synchrony of the CMAP (Fig. 4–7), but these changes lag behind clinical recovery and may take many months to return to normal. In fact, complete return to normal may not occur in severe cases, even when excellent functional recovery occurs, presumably because of the increased number of nodes of Ranvier, and therefore increased summated nodal delay, associated with remyelination.

Physiological Basis for Symptoms in GBS

Studies of antiserum-induced demyelination in experimental animals has provided insights into the physiological basis for the observed clinical deficits in patients with GBS.[25] Perhaps most importantly, they have provided an explanation for observation that nerve conduction studies often appear worse as the patient improves. Twenty-four hours after injection of demyelinating antiserum into the sciatic nerve, recipient rats are severely weak in sciatic innervated muscles. At that time distal conduction is normal but there is focal conduction block at the site of demyelination. By analogy, patients with GBS may be severely weak and yet have normal distal conduction studies. The weakness results from conduction block at more proximal sites as demonstrated by Mills and Murray.[26] Furthermore, Berger et al.[27] found that recovery of strength coincided with return of previously absent F-waves, even while distal conduction remained entirely unchanged. Conversely, with antiserum-induced demyelination, complete clinical recovery occurs at the time when the most dramatic changes in nerve conduction are seen. During the second week, rats are clinically normal and yet severe slowing of maximal conduction velocity and profound dispersion of the proximal CMAP remains. This indicates that conduction slowing and desynchrony of propagated electrical potentials do not result in any significant clinical abnormality. Thus, the patient with severe paralysis from GBS may have singularly unimpressive nerve conduction changes, limited to impersistent F-waves and low amplitude distal motor responses, during the first week or so of illness. A month later, the same patient may be almost fully recovered and yet have severe conduction slowing and marked temporal dispersion of evoked responses. A second observation made in experimental demyelination is that the small diameter axons are more susceptible to demyelinative conduction block than larger ones. This suggests that the early reflex loss may be caused by conduction block in smaller diameter fusimotor efferent fibers rather than in the largest type Ia afferents, as is usually suggested. Third, these studies provide at least a partial explanation for the distribution of demyelinative lesions in GBS. The perineurim in the sciatic nerve provides an effective barrier to diffusion of antiserum into the endoneurium whereas ventral nerve roots are highly permeable. This may explain the predilection for GBS to attack nerve roots early. Blood–nerve barrier is also relatively deficient at axon branch points, which may account for the early involvement of intramuscular motor nerves.

Nerve Conduction Studies in GBS

Nerve conduction studies provide the most specific evidence of focal or multifocal demyelination and remyelination in GBS and are abnormal at some time during the evolution of the disease in almost all patients. As previously mentioned, the distribution of pathological lesions is not random (Table 4–1). In the earliest phase of the disease, foci of demyelination are concentrated in nerve roots, particularly ventral roots. Involvement of distal intramuscular nerves at their branch points and areas of nerve prone to compression (carpal tunnel, cubital tunnel, etc.) is seen next. Finally, as the disease progresses, patchy demyelination is usually seen along the length of nerve trunks. It should be stressed that individual patients or individual nerves may diverge from this general pattern. Nonetheless, it follows that early nerve conduction studies should concentrate on the most proximal and most distal nerve segments. Although the pathological lesions in GBS ultimately become widely and bilaterally distributed, early in the course of the disease the degree of involvement may differ markedly from nerve to nerve and from side to side so multiple nerves should be studied in all four limbs and, if clinically indicated, in the muscles innervated by cranial nerves. The importance of studying multiple nerves is demonstrated by three recent studies[9,16,28] of more than 1000 nerves in 305 patients in which only 1 patient was normal, even though most had only a single study. By contrast, earlier studies that had reported a much higher incidence of negative results, ranging from 14% to 41%, were single studies and involved only a few nerves.[29-33] In the most recent of his two studies of patients in whom a single electrodiagnostic evaluation was done, McLeod found normal conduction is some of the nerves studied in 30% of the patients whereas only 9% of patients had normal conduction in all nerves studied.[34]

Several investigators[8-11] have attempted to develop electrodiagnostic criteria to quantitate the changes of acute demyelination. These are useful

Table 4–1. Hierarchy of Susceptibility to Demyelination in GBS

1. Nerve roots (particularly ventral)
2. Intramuscular motor axons
3. Sites prone to compression
4. Nerve trunks

as a guide for electrodiagnosticians and are even more important as a means of ensuring uniformity in multicenter experimental studies. The extremely sensitive criteria suggested by Albers et al.[9] are impractical for routine use in the diagnosis of GBS since they would encompass a significant number of patients without other evidence of the demyelination if applied without taking other diagnostic features into account. Albers[10] later relaxed these criteria but even the more recent criteria are relatively nonspecific and carry a significant risk of including patients without GBS if applied injudiciously. More stringent velocity criteria were suggested by Kelly,[8] but no quantitation of criteria for distal motor latency, F-wave latency, or conduction block were given. The criteria suggested by Cornblath[11] are more specific but will undoubtedly exclude some patients who meet the clinical criteria for the diagnosis of GBS. Each of these sets of criteria has been developed to assist in the recognition of acute demyelination and should be used, along with the other diagnostic criteria, to support a diagnosis of GBS. If they are injudiciously applied without knowledge of the clinical features and the CSF picture, individual patients will be misdiagnosed and may receive inappropriate and not entirely benign treatment or may be excluded from receiving necessary treatment.

Motor Nerve Conduction Studies

Abnormalities of motor nerve conduction almost always exceed sensory changes. Albers et al.[9] found some form of abnormal motor conduction in 96% of 70 patients in whom serial studies were done. At the time of the first study 88% were abnormal and the peak abnormalities were found 3 weeks into the illness, although not all abnormalities fulfilled electrodiagnostic criteria for demyelination. In 10% of patients, the results had some features suggestive of demyelination but were classified overall as indeterminate, whereas a further 3% showed the features of axonal degeneration only. The changes most specific for demyelination are focal conduction block and focal temporal dispersion, but these abnormalities can be established with certainty in only a minority of cases, at least early in the evolution of the disease process. Similarly, Ropper et al. found some abnormality of motor conduction in about 90% of patients.[16]

F-WAVE ABNORMALITIES

In keeping with the distribution of pathology, the earliest and most prominent abnormalities are found proximally and distally. Kimura[35,36] studied F-wave conduction velocity in the median and ulnar nerves in patients with mild GBS. In their initial small study of nine patients, they found that proximal conduction was more often slowed than distal and suggested that F-wave velocity determination was useful in the early diagnosis of GBS. They later studied 126 arm nerves in 45 patients with GBS and found that about half of the patients had slowing in both proximal and distal segments. In the other half, slowing was accentuated either proximally or distally in almost exactly equal numbers. Walsh et al.[37] studied median F-waves after wrist stimulation in 17 patients with GBS and found that they were abnormal in only 8, and in 6 of these the distal conduction studies were also abnormal. Conversely, in three patients with abnormal distal conduction the F-waves were normal. Olney and Aminoff[38] studied median, ulnar, and peroneal F-waves in 15 patients (44 nerves) with GBS. Peripheral motor conduction was abnormal in 33 of 44 nerves and the F-wave was abnormal in 31. In eight nerves, distal motor conduction was abnormal but F-waves were normal whereas in six nerves F-waves were abnormal with normal distal motor conduction. Ropper et al.[16] found that the two most common abnormalities were "proximal conduction block" alone (27%), which they defined as absent F-waves, and proximal block plus distal motor conduction abnormality (27%). Abnormal conduction in the intermediate nerve segments is less frequent and generally occurs later. None of these reports addresses the paradox of a normal F-wave latency when distal conduction is slowed. There is general agreement among these and other authors[39–41] that the F-wave may be abnormal in a proportion of patients with GBS in whom other electrophysiological parameters are normal. As such, they may provide clues to an otherwise uncertain diagnosis, especially early in the course of the disease. We have found that, although either impersistent F-waves or prolonged F-wave latencies (Fig. 4–2) may be the only abnormality in a single nerve, other nerves in the same patient have other abnormalities in intermediate or distal segments. Therefore, in isolation, F-wave abnormalities should be interpreted with caution since there are usually widespread multifocal, electrophysiological abnormalities.

MOTOR NERVE CONDUCTION

The characteristic features of conduction block, conduction slowing, and differential temporal dispersion of CMAPs have already been described and are shown in Figures 4–3 and 4–7. Although the changes are often found in a patchy distribution, they almost invariably become widespread in time, involving most nerves and nerve segments to some extent. However, although motor nerve conduction studies are almost invariably abnormal in GBS, they do not always meet the criteria for demyelination in patients who meet the other National Institute of Neurological and Communicative Disorders and Stroke (NINCDS) criteria for the diagnosis of GBS. Ten percent of the patients in Albers's series had features of axonal degeneration and in 3%, there was pure axonal degeneration.[10] In addition, a severe, pure axonal form of acute neuropathy, perhaps akin to GBS, has been described. Feasby et al.[42] described five patients in whom all motor nerves were inexcitable and subsequently all patients developed widespread fibrillation on needle electromyography (EMG). At autopsy, one patient had widespread axonal degeneration without demyelination or inflammation. Miller et al.[43] described a clinically similar but electrophysiologically more heterogeneous syndrome. Some motor nerves were inexcitable whereas others had responses of extremely low amplitude and all patients went on to develop profuse fibrillation on needle EMG. Motor conduction velocity, when it could be recorded, was only moderately slowed, consistent with loss of the fastest conducting axons. They invoke lesions confined to the most distal motor nerve segments to explain the findings, based on the very early appearance of inexcitable nerves, normal conduction in adjacent sensory nerves, and prolongation in the distal motor latency in those cases in which it could be recorded. However, the poor recovery in all of their patients militates against lesions confined to a distal site. Numerous other reports attest to occasional severe axonal degeneration in GBS but in most it is accompanied by prominent demyelination.[44-47]

In addition to the routine limb nerve studies, motor conduction studies of the phrenic nerve are often abnormal in GBS.[48,49] Gourie-Devi and Ganapathy[49] found abnormal phrenic conduction in 64% of their GBS patients and claimed that it was more accurate than other nerve conduction studies or even vital capacity for predicting respiratory failure.

Sensory Nerve Conduction Studies

Abnormalities of sensory conduction are almost as common as motor but they are not as helpful diagnostically. In his serial studies, Albers[10] found abnormal sensory conduction in 83% of patients between the sixth and tenth weeks of illness. However, during the first week of illness sensory conduction was abnormal in only 25% of patients, increasing to 73% by the third week. Ropper et al.[16] found abnormalities of sensory conduction in only 62% of patients tested on a single occasion during the first 3 weeks of the illness whereas McLeod[33] reported 76% of patients had abnormal sensory conduction, findings closely comparable to those of Albers. Loss of the sensory potentials in the face of normal motor conduction has been reported in patients with Miller-Fisher syndrome.[50] The relative paucity of sensory conduction abnormalities partly reflects the predilection of the disease for nerve roots but even when comparable segments of motor nerves are severely involved the sensory studies may remain normal. The earliest changes, when they do occur, may involve the shape of the wave form, which is seldom closely analyzed in clinical electrodiagnostic studies. Since antibody-induced demyelination does not initially involve the largest myelinated axons, maximal sensory conduction velocity may be normal but the normally compact sensory nerve action potential (SNAP) develops slight dispersion of its late components, which is likely to be missed without prolonged signal averaging. Frank dispersion may be seen as demyelination progresses if many responses are computer averaged. However, the usual change with routine studies is for the SNAP amplitude to decrease as a result of conduction block in some sensory fibers and phase cancellation of others associated with the dispersion. Some slowing of sensory conduction velocity is seen but it seldom is profound since the SNAP usually disappears before severe slowing supervenes.

H-reflexes

The H-reflex, unlike the F-wave, measures the passage of electrical impulses through a reflex arc involving both sensory and motor fibers. It can be recorded only in a limited number of muscles in normal humans and is most frequently studied in the triceps surae complex. If the F-wave recorded from the peroneal or tibial nerves is abnormal, the H-reflex should also be abnormal since the efferent component of the H-reflex traverses the same pathway as the F-wave. However, if the F-wave is normal, abnormalities of the H-reflex latency indicate an abnormality in the proximal, peripheral sensory pathway. If the Achilles tendon reflex is unobtainable, the H-reflex is also usually absent since it is no more than the electrophysiological manifestation of this clinical reflex. Since the Achilles tendon reflex is usually lost in GBS, this limits the usefulness of the H-reflex in evaluating proximal segments of the sensory nerves. Furthermore, since the H-reflex may be occasionally absent in normal individuals, its absence in suspected GBS is not necessarily abnormal. Nonetheless, prolongation of the H-reflex latency was found to be the most common abnormality of tibial nerve conduction in one study of 23 GBS patients.[51]

Blink Reflexes

The blink reflex can be used to assess conduction in a cranial reflex arc involving the fifth (afferent) and seventh (efferent) cranial nerves. Stimulation of the supraorbital branch of the trigeminal nerve produces a short latency ipsilateral response from facial muscles as well as a longer latency bilateral response. The facial nerve may be involved in as many as 50% of patients with GBS and it is not surprising that the blink reflex is abnormal in these cases, showing conduction block or slowing.[16] The blink reflex may also be abnormal in those cases where early involvement is confined to cranial nerves such as Miller-Fisher syndrome, even when the facial and trigeminal nerves are not overtly involved.[52,53] It is also useful in patients with coincident neuropathies, such as diabetic neuropathy, where the limb nerves may have severe preexisting changes that mask the superimposed demyelinative changes of GBS.[54] The blink reflex is seldom affected in axonal neuropathies and abnormalities in this reflex arc may provide an important clue to otherwise covert demyelination.[55]

Evoked Potentials

Somatosensory evoked potentials (SSEPs) can be used to unearth covert abnormalities of conduction in proximal segments of peripheral nerves as well as the dorsal roots. Walsh et al.[37] found that there was a higher yield of abnormality using SSEPs than with either motor nerve conduction studies or F-waves. They studied only the median nerve and found that SSEPs were abnormal in five of their six patients with normal F-waves and in three of the six patients in whom all other electrophysiological studies were normal. However, Olney and Aminoff[38] studied median, ulnar, and peroneal nerves and found that only 5 of 11 patients had abnormal SSEPs while the F-waves were abnormal in 9. Only one patient had abnormal SSEPs with normal F-waves and this patient had abnormal distal sensory responses. Gilmore and Nelson[41] studied SSEPs and F-waves in the median and tibial nerves in patients with GBS within 2 weeks of the onset of symptoms. At this relatively early stage of the disease, 10 of 18 patients had abnormal median SSEPs and 17 of 19 had abnormal tibial SSEPs. By comparison, 16 of 18 had abnormal median F-waves and 12 of 19 had abnormal tibial F-waves. A frequent abnormality was the complete absence of the SSEP at all sites of recording, suggesting the presence of conduction block in sensory axons. Absence of the SSEP recorded from Erb's point or lumbar or cervical spine could be attributed to dispersion of the electrical potential related to conduction slowing but, in such cases, a cortical response can still be recorded, even when the peripheral sensory conduction velocity is as slow as 18 m/s.[56] Several other reports[57,58] have also attested to the ability of SSEPs to detect abnormal, proximal sensory conduction when other studies remain normal. They therefore appear to have a role in confirming a suspected diagnosis in those occasional cases when more traditional nerve conduction studies are normal. However, they add little to the routine evaluation of GBS.

Although rarely involved clinically, the auditory nerve is not immune from demyelination in GBS. Therefore, brainstem auditory evoked responses (BAER) may be abnormal. Schiff et al.[59] reported four of five patients with abnormal interpeak latencies, primarily between peaks I and III, thought to be due to retrocochlear demyelination causing slowing of conduction velocity in the acoustic nerve. However, Ropper and Chiappa[57] found that only 3 of 21 GBS patients had abnormal BAERs and none of the 3 patients reported by Jamal and Ballantyne[60] was abnormal. Nelson et al.[61] report two patients with temporary hearing loss associated with GBS. In one, there was complete loss of all BAER waveforms suggesting acute conduction block in the acoustic nerve. During convalescence, hearing recovered and the BAER returned but with profoundly slowed peripheral conduction velocity (prolonged wave I latency). The second patient did not have conduction block but did have marked slowing of peripheral conduction velocity. There have been occasional reports of abnormal conduction in central pathways, usually in patients with Miller-Fisher syndrome.[62,63] However, the reports have been sporadic and do not provide strong support for the hypothesis that Miller-Fisher syndrome is accompanied by a brain stem encephalitis.

Papilledema is seen in about 5% of patients with GBS and causes abnormalities of the visual evoked potential (VEP).[57] Similarly, optic neuritis rarely complicates GBS and causes loss of the VEP. However, the VEP has rarely been studied in uncomplicated cases of GBS. In those instances in which it has been reported it has been normal.[53] Thus, there is no evidence of subclinical involvement of visual pathways in the usual cases of GBS.

Magnetic Stimulation

Since ventral nerve roots bear the primary brunt of demyelination in GBS, much effort has been directed toward studying proximal conduction using the indirect methods of F-wave and H-reflex conduction times. SSEPs provide a more direct measure of proximal conduction velocity but have two major disadvantages. First, the sensory pathways are often relatively spared. Second, with SSEPs, conduction is measured over long nerve segments and the effect of slow conduction velocity over a few centimeters of the nerve root segment may be diluted by normal conduction velocity along the meter or so of the rest of the peripheral nerve pathway. Magnetic stimulation appeared to offer an opportunity to study nerve conduction in proximal segments more directly. The depolarizing current generated by an electromagnetic coil is not significantly attenuated by increasing distance from the coil or by the nature of intervening tissues.[64] Stimulation of cortex through bone or peripheral nerves through clothing was found to be quite feasible. This led to the hope that nerves anatomically situated a considerable distance from the skin could be supramaximally stimulated, which would have made magnetic stimulation an ideal tool for directly studying proximal nerves and nerve roots in GBS. Unfortunately, at its present stage of development, two drawbacks have limited its applicability. First, it has proved difficult to stimulate deeply located nerves supramaximally and second, it is impossible to localize accurately the site at which the nerve is being depolarized.[65-67] At its current stage of development, these technical factors have made it impossible to evaluate either conduction velocity or conduction block accurately and has drastically limited its usefulness in the electrodiagnostic evaluation of GBS.

Needle EMG in GBS

Whereas the nerve conduction studies are invaluable in the diagnosis of GBS, needle EMG is used primarily in prognosis. However, the EMG can provide evidence of proximal demyelination in cases where the distal conduction studies are normal or equivocal. When there is partial conduction block confined to the most proximal segments of motor nerves, the distally elicited compound muscle action potential will be of normal amplitude. When a needle electrode is inserted into the same muscle, there will be no spontaneous activity at rest and motor unit potentials will have a normal appearance. However, motor unit recruitment will be abnormal with rapid firing of individual motor units and a reduced maximal interference pattern. In addition, the presence of demyelination may be inferred by surface recording of motor unit recruitment. With volitional contraction of the muscle the surface recorded motor units may be used to "synthesize" a compound muscle action potential.[19] If this reconstituted CMAP does not closely resemble the electrically elicited response, proximal conduction block may be inferred. This technique can be useful when there are only a few motor units under volitional control but requires full cooperation of the patient.

Facial myokymia is relatively commonly seen in GBS and is occasionally also seen in limb muscles.[68–71] In one study, myokymia was seen clinically and confirmed electromyographically in 17% of 48 consecutive GBS patients.[68] The myokymia is usually seen within the first week of the illness but may persist for up to 6 weeks. It usually is confined to weak muscles. Fasciculations are rarely seen clinically but may be seen with needle EMG during the first few weeks of the illness.

Autonomic Testing in GBS

Autonomic instability has become a major cause of morbidity and mortality of GBS as ventilator technology has advanced. A number of reports have detailed a variety of objective abnormalities of autonomic function as outlined in Chapter 2. However, there have been no studies of the predictive value of abnormalities of autonomic testing. It would be useful to have an objective test or group of tests whereby those patients at risk for developing serious autonomic instability could be identified and monitored appropriately.

Prognosis and Prognostic Indicators

GBS usually is a monophasic illness and complete or partial recovery is to be expected. In their retrospective study of 40 patients collected from a 42-year period, Kennedy et al.[72] found that recovery, as judged by return to all former activities, was complete in 31 and partial in 7 patients who survived the acute illness. Andersson and Siden[73] found a similar high rate of recovery with 54 out of 56 survivors making a complete functional recovery; 30% within 3 months, 73% within 6 months, and the remainder by 18 months. Several other studies[74–77] have reported complete functional recovery in more than 75% of cases. In contrast, McLeod et al.[33] found that less than 50% of 18 patients recovered completely although only 4 had significant disability. The difference probably relates to differences in data collection. The larger epidemiological studies rely more on patient reports of recovery or retrospective evaluation of medical records. McLeod et al. examined their patients prospectively and documented mild abnormalities of neurological examination such as absent ankle reflexes and impaired two-point discrimination, abnormalities that are unlikely to have functional significance. Although there is general agreement that excellent recovery occurs in more patients with GBS, about 15% of survivors are left with a significant disability.

Clinical Predictors of Outcome

Several studies have sought to identify factors that might enable a prediction of outcome at the time of the acute illness. It has been suggested that CSF pleocytosis,[78] severe sensory loss or a prolonged progressive phase,[77,79] and papilledema[80] all carry an ominous prognosis. However, others[81–85] have disputed these claims. Winer et al.[86] and Miller et al.[85] found that the most powerful and reliable clinical predictor of poor outcome was the need for ventilator assistance during the acute illness, and Ravn[76] and Loffel et al.[77] noted that severe maximum motor impairment, not surprisingly, carried a poorer prognosis. Some authors have stressed that children have a significantly higher incidence of permanent and significant neurological sequelae,[76,86] although more recent studies have not confirmed this.[88,89] In fact, a recent study found that not only did children have a better prognosis than adults but the electrophysiological prognostic indicators in children did not carry such an ominous outlook.[89] Paradoxically, even those studies that showed greater peak disability and permanent sequelae in children found that mortality is lower.[86,90]

Electrophysiological Predictors of Outcome

The most important determinant of rate and efficacy of recovery is the degree of axonal degeneration that accompanies the demyelination. Remyelination is an efficient and rapid process that is usually completed within 4 to 6 months of the nadir of the illness. Thus, even severe neurological disability resulting solely from demyelination may recover completely within a few months of the onset of disease. Conversely, axonal regeneration is a slow and inefficient process, with elongation of regenerating sprouts occurring at a rate of less than 1 mm/day. Therefore, recovery occurs over many months and may not be maximal for up to 2 years. Furthermore, even if regeneration occurs, the axon may fail to make synaptic contact with an appropriate receptor or effector organ so functional recovery fails. Additionally, synaptic contact may be made with inappropriate end organs (aberrant regeneration), resulting in abnormal function that may be worse than lack of function.

The most reliable overall predictors of axonal degeneration and therefore of outcome in GBS are the nerve conduction studies and EMG. Miller et al.,[85] Cornblath et al.,[91] McKhann et al.,[92] and Ropper et al.[16] all found that a low amplitude CMAP, even when recorded during the early stages of the disease, carried an ominous prognosis. In the former study, 60 patients who were bedfast, 22 of whom were ventilator dependent, were analyzed retrospectively to see which factors correlated significantly with their poor recovery. The only electrophysiological parameter that correlated significantly was the low CMAP amplitude. They found no significant correlation between poor outcome and density of fibrillation potentials found with needle EMG. The studies of Cornblath et al. and McKhann et al. report the results of the North American multicenter trial of plasmapheresis for GBS, in which no needle EMG data were gathered. Again, the only significant correlation with poor outcome was low amplitude CMAP. However, even in those patients in whom the CMAP amplitude was 0% to 20% of normal, outcome was still improved with plasmapheresis more than those patients who received no treatment.

Pleasure et al.[83] were the first to suggest that the presence of fibrillation potentials in weak muscles at the nadir of weakness predicted a poor outcome. Their observations were confirmed in more extensive studies by Eisen and Humphries,[32] McLeod et al.[33] and Raman and Taori.[84] However, neither Miller et al.[85] nor Ropper et al.[16] found any correlation between fibrillations and outcome, independent of CMAP amplitude. For example, Ropper et al. found widespread fibrillation in 10 of 113 patients, most of whom were studied in the first 3 weeks of illness. However, only those two patients in whom the CMAP amplitude was also severely reduced failed to make complete recovery.

Since recovery depends primarily on the degree of axonal degeneration, it is hardly surprising that patients with electrodiagnostic evidence of severe axonal degeneration should have a worse outcome. Fibrillation of muscle indicates loss of the trophic influence of axons on muscle fibers due to axonal degeneration. A low amplitude CMAP may also be due to acute axonal degeneration. Conduction block in distal intramuscular nerve twigs can give the same result, although the CMAP is usually dispersed and the distal motor latency prolonged. However, in individual patients it is wise not to make ominous predictions too confidently, based on low amplitude CMAP in a single study. This point was underscored by Triggs et al.,[93] who found that of eight patients with inexcitable motor nerves at the time of the initial study, only three had severe residual disability at 12 months. The remainder had improved significantly at 3 months and had recovered completely by 12 months. They emphasize the importance of sequential studies before confident predictions can be made. Nonetheless, if the amplitude is reduced to less than 10% of normal, regardless of whether it is initially due to severe conduction block or axonal degeneration, the end result tends to be severe axonal degeneration and carries a poor prognosis.

Designing an Electrophysiologic Study for GBS

Electrophysiologic studies in GBS fall into two categories: diagnostic and prognostic. The diagnosis of GBS is primarily based on the nerve conduction studies (NCS) whereas prognostication relies on both NCS and needle EMG. In the interest of timely diagnosis, NCS should be performed as soon as possible. However, the earliest studies may appear normal or at least may not establish a certain diagnosis. More important than the findings of a single study is to demonstrate the evolution of the characteristic electrodiagnostic changes, as set out above. Multiple motor nerves should be studied, concentrating on nerves innervating clinically weak muscles. In addition, multiple segments of each nerve should be studied when feasible; for example, in the arms, the median or ulnar nerve should be stimulated at the wrist, elbow, axilla, and perhaps Erb's point. The CMAP amplitude should be recorded for each stimulus site and each waveform carefully examined for early dispersion. F-waves should be recorded for each motor nerve and the minimum latency and percentage of F-wave firings noted. Sensory nerve conduction studies are mainly useful in a negative sense. They are usually only mildly abnormal and the changes are nonspecific; severe abnormalities of sensory nerve conduction should raise questions about a diagnosis of GBS. Similarly, the needle EMG is of limited use diagnostically.

If the initial electrodiagnostic study is equivocal it should be repeated 1 to 5 days later, depending on the severity of the paralysis. Once the nadir of the illness has been reached, studies should be repeated and should include needle EMG of both distal and proximal muscles to determine the severity and distribution of any denervation, again concentrating on the weaker muscles. Paraspinal muscles should be studied since significant denervation at this level indicates axonal degeneration involving ventral nerve roots, which augurs poorly for functional recovery in muscles of the affected segments. Additional useful prognostic information may sometimes be obtained by repeating the needle EMG over subsequent months to follow the process of reinnervation by regeneration.

Summary

The electrodiagnostic studies provide critical diagnostic and prognostic information in GBS and have replaced CSF examination as the most important investigation in patients with acutely evolving paralysis. They have also provided considerable insight into the pathophysiology of demyelination and have furthered our understanding of the physiological basis of the symptoms and signs in GBS.

References

1. McDonald WI. The effects of experimental demyelination on conduction in peripheral nerve: a histological and electrophysiological study. II. Electrophysiological observations. *Brain.* 1963;86:501–524.
2. Dyck PJ, Lambert EH. Lower motor and primary sensory neuron diseases with peroneal muscular atrophy. *Arch Neurol.* 1968;18:603–618.
3. Buchthal F, Behse F. Peroneal muscular atrophy (PMA) and related disorders. I. Clinical manifestations as related to biopsy findings, nerve conduction and electromyography. *Brain.* 1977;100:41–66.
4. Gilliatt RW. Nerve conduction in human and experimental neuropathies. *Proc Roy Soc Med.* 1966;59:989–993.
5. Cragg BG, Thomas PK. Changes in nerve conduction in experimental allergic neuritis. *J Neurol Neurosurg Psychiatry.* 1964;27:106–115.
6. Brown WF, Feasby TE. Conduction block and denervation in Guillain-Barré polyneuropathy. *Brain.* 1984;107:219–239.
7. Feasby TE, Brown WF, Gilbert JJ, Hahn AF. The pathological basis of conduction block in human neuropathies. *J Neurol Neurosurg Psychiatry.* 1985;43:239–244.

8. Kelly JJ. The electrodiagnostic findings in the peripheral neuropathy associated with monoclonal gammopathy. *Muscle Nerve*. 1983;6:504–509.
9. Albers JW, Donofrio PD, McGonagle TK. Sequential electrodiagnostic abnormalities in acute inflammatory demyelinating polyradiculoneuropathy. *Muscle Nerve*. 1985;8:528–539.
10. Albers JW. AAEE case report #4: Guillain-Barré syndrome. *Muscle Nerve*. 1989;12:705–711.
11. Cornblath DR. Electrophysiology in Guillain-Barré syndrome. *Ann Neurol*. 1990;27(suppl): S17–S20.
12. Saida K, Saida T, Brown MJ, Silberberg DH, Asbury AK. Antiserum-mediated demyelination in vivo. A sequential study using intraneural injection of experimental allergic neuritis serum. *Lab Invest*. 1978;39:449–462.
13. Sumner AJ, Saida K, Saida T, Silberberg DH, Asbury AK. Acute conduction block associated with experimental antiserum-mediated demyelination of peripheral nerve. *Ann Neurol*. 1982; 11:469–477.
14. LaFontaine S, Rasminsky M, Saida T, Sumner AJ. Conduction block in rat myelinated fibres following acute exposure to anti-galactocerebroside serum. *J Physiol*. 1982;323:287–306.
15. Kimura J, Butzer JF. F-wave conduction velocity in Guillain-Barré syndrome. Assessment of nerve segment between axilla and spinal cord. *Arch Neurol*. 1975;32:524–529.
16. Ropper AH, Wijdicks EFM, Shahani BT. Electrodiagnostic abnormalities in 113 consecutive patients with Guillain-Barré syndrome. *Arch Neurol*. 1990;47:881–887.
17. Lewis RA, Sumner AJ, Brown MJ, Asbury AK. Multifocal demyelinating neuropathy with persistent conduction block. *Neurology*. 1982;32:958–964.
18. Rhee EK, Englan JD, Sumner AJ. A computer simulation of conduction block: effects produced by actual block versus interphase cancellation. *Ann Neurol*. 1990;28:146–156.
19. Sumner AJ. Separating motor neuron diseases from pure motor neuropathies. Multifocal motor neuropathy with persistent conduction block. *Adv Neurol*. 1991;56:399–403.
20. Krarup C, Steward JD, Sumner AJ, Pestronk A, Lipton SA. A syndrome of asymmetric limb weakness with motor conduction block. *Neurology*. 1990;40:118–127.
21. Trojaberg W, Lange DL, Latov N, Younger DS, Lovelace RE, Rowland LP. Conduction block and other abnormalities of nerve conduction in motor neuron disease: a review of 110 patients. *Neurology*. 1990;40(suppl 1):182.
22. Cornblath DR, Sumner AJ, Daube J, et al. Conduction block in clinical practice. *Muscle Nerve*. 1991;14:869–871.
23. Rasminsky M. Pathophysiology of demyelination. *Ann NY Acad Sci*. 1984;436:68–85.
24. Saida K, Sumner AJ, Saida T, Brown MJ, Silberberg DH. Antiserum-mediated demyelination: relationship between remyelination and functional recovery. *Ann Neurol*. 1980;8:12–24.
25. Sumner AJ. The physiological basis for symptoms in Guillain-Barré syndrome. *Ann Neurol*. 1980;9(suppl):28–30.
26. Mills KR, Murray NMF. Proximal conduction block in early Guillain-Barré syndrome. *Lancet*. 1985;2:659.
27. Berger AR, Logigian EL, Shahani BT. Reversible proximal conduction block underlies rapid recovery in Guillain-Barré syndrome. *Muscle Nerve*. 1988;11:1039–1042.
28. Thomas TD, Oh SJ, Bosse B, Joy J. Diagnostic sensitivity of the initial nerve conduction study in acute inflammatory demyelinating polyneuropathy. *Neurology*. 1991;41:(suppl 1):132. Abstract.
29. Lambert EH, Mulder DW. Nerve conduction in the Guillain-Barré syndrome. *Electroencephalogr Clin Neurophysiol*. 1964;17:86. Abstract.
30. Bergamini L, Gandiglio G, Fra L. Motor and afferent nerve conduction in the Guillain-Barré syndrome. *Electromyography*. 1966;6:205–232.
31. McQuillen MP. Idiopathic polyneuritis: serial studies of nerve and immune functions. *J Neurol Neurosurg Psychiatry*. 1971;34:607–615.
32. Eisen A, Humphreys P. The Guillain-Barré syndrome. A clinical and electrodiagnostic study of 25 cases. *Arch Neurol*. 1974;30:438–443.
33. McLeod JG, Walsh JC, Prineas JW, Pollard JG. Acute idiopathic polyneuritis: a clinical and electrophysiological follow-up study. *J Neurol Sci*. 1976;27:145–162.
34. McLeod JG. Electrophysiological studies in the Guillain-Barré syndrome. *Ann Neurol*. 1981;9(suppl):20–27.
35. Kimura J. F-wave velocity in the central segment of the median and ulnar nerves. A study in normal subjects and in patients with Charcot-Marie-Tooth disease. *Neurology*. 1974;24:539–546.
36. Kimura J. Proximal versus distal slowing of motor nerve conduction velocity in the Guillain-Barré syndrome. *Ann Neurol*. 1978;3:344–350.

37. Walsh JC, Yiannikas C, McLeod JG. Abnormalities of proximal conduction in acute idiopathic polyneuritis: comparison of short latency evoked potentials and F-waves. *J Neurol Neurosurg Psychiatry*. 1984;47:197–200.
38. Olney RK, Aminoff MJ. Electrodiagnostic features of the Guillain-Barré syndrome: the relative sensitivity of different techniques. *Neurology*. 1990;40:471–475.
39. King D, Ashby P. Conduction velocity in the proximal segments of a motor nerve in the Guillain-Barré syndrome. *J Neurol Neurosurg Psychiatry*. 1976;39:538–544.
40. Lachman T, Shahani BT, Young RR. Late responses as aids to diagnosis in peripheral neuropathy. *J Neurol Neurosurg Psychiatry*. 1980;43:156–162.
41. Gilmore RL, Nelson KR. SSEP and F-wave studies in acute inflammatory demyelinating polyradiculoneuropathy. *Muscle Nerve*. 1989;12:538–543.
42. Feasby TE, Gilbert JJ, Brown WF, et al. An acute axonal form of Guillain-Barré polyneuropathy. *Brain*. 1986;109:1115–1126.
43. Miller RG, Peterson C, Rosenberg NL. Electrophysiologic evidence of severe distal nerve segment pathology in the Guillain-Barré syndrome. *Muscle Nerve*. 1987;10:524–529.
44. Haymaker W, Kernohan JW. The Landry-Guillain-Barré syndrome. A clinicopathological report of fifty fatal cases and a critique of the literature. *Medicine*. 1949;28:59–141.
45. Asbury AK, Arnason BG, Adams RD. The inflammatory lesion in idiopathic polyneuritis: its role in the pathogenesis. *Medicine*. 1969;48:173–215.
46. Feasby TE, Hahn AF, Gilbert JJ. Passive transfer studies in Guillain-Barré polyneuropathy. *Neurology*. 1982;32:1159–1167.
47. Vallat JM, Hugon J, Tabaraud F, Leboutet MJ, Chazot F, Dumas M. Quatre cas de syndrome de Guillain-Barré avec lesions axonales. *Rev Neurol*. 1990;146:420–424.
48. Newsom-Davies J. Phrenic nerve conduction in man. *J Neurol Neurosurg Psychiatry*. 1967; 30:420–426.
49. Gourie-Devi M, Ganapathy GR. Phrenic nerve conduction time in Guillain-Barré syndrome. *J Neurol Neurosurg Psychiatry*. 1985;48:245–249.
50. Guiloff RJ. Peripheral nerve conduction in Miller Fisher syndrome. *J Neurol Neurosurg Psychiatry*. 1977;40:801–807.
51. Takeuchi H, Takahashi M, Kang J, et al. The Guillain-Barré syndrome: Clinical and electroneurographic studies. *J Neurol*. 1984;231:6–10.
52. Fross RD, Daube JR. Neuropathy in the Miller Fisher syndrome: clinical and electrophysiological findings. *Neurology*. 1987;37:1493–1498.
53. Jamal GA, MacLeod WN. Electrophysiologic studies in Miller Fisher syndrome. *Neurology*. 1984;34:685–688.
54. Kimura J. An evaluation of the facial and trigeminal nerves in polyneuropathy: electrodiagnostic study in Charcot-Marie-Tooth disease, Guillain-Barré syndrome and diabetic neuropathy. *Neurology*. 1971;21:747–753.
55. Ropper AH, Shahani BT. Diagnosis and management of acute arelexic paralysis with emphasis on Guillain-Barré syndrome. In: Asbury AK, Gilliatt RW, eds. *Peripheral nerve disorders*. London: Butterworths; 1984:21–45.
56. Parry GJ, Aminoff MJ. Somatosensory evoked potentials in chronic acquired demyelinating peripheral neuropathy. *Neurology*. 1987;37:313–316.
57. Ropper AH, Chiappa KH. Evoked potentials in Guillain-Barré syndrome. *Neurology*. 1986;36:587–590.
58. Ganji S, Frazier E. Somatosensory evoked potential studies in acute Guillain-Barré syndrome. *Electromyogr Clin Neurophysiol*. 1988;28:313–317.
59. Schiff JA, Cracco RQ, Cracco JB. Brainstem auditory evoked potentials in Guillain-Barré syndrome. *Neurology*. 1985;35:771–773.
60. Jamal GA, Ballantyne JP. The localization of the lesion in patients with acute ophthalmoplegia, ataxia and areflexia (Miller Fisher syndrome). A serial multimodal neurophysiological study. *Brain*. 1988;111:95–114.
61. Nelson KR, Gilmore RL, Massey A. Acoustic nerve conduction abnormalities in Guillain-Barré syndrome. *Neurology*. 1988;38:1263–1266.
62. Al-Din AM, Anderson M, Bickerstaff ER, Harvey I. Brainstem encephalitis and the syndrome of Miller Fisher. A clinical study. *Brain*. 1982;105:481–495.
63. Rudolph SH, Montesinos C, Shanzer S. Abnormal brainstem auditory evoked potentials in Fisher syndrome. *Neurology*. 1985;35(suppl 1):70.
64. Barker AT, Jalinous R, Freeston IL. Non-invasive stimulation of the human motor cortex. *Lancet*. 1985;1:1106–1107.

65. Evans BA, Daube JR, Litchy WJ. A comparison of magnetic and electrical stimulation of spinal nerves. *Muscle Nerve*. 1990;13:414–420.
66. Olney RK, So YT, Goodin DS, Aminoff MJ. A comparison of magnetic and electrical stimulation of peripheral nerves. *Muscle Nerve*. 1990;13:957–963.
67. Cros D, Day TJ, Shahani BT. Spatial dispersion of stimulation in peripheral nerves. *Muscle Nerve*. 1990;13:1076–1082.
68. Mateer JE, Gutmann L, McComas CF. Myokymia in Guillain-Barré syndrome. *Neurology*. 1983;33:374–376.
69. Wasserstrom WR, Starr A. Facial myokymia in the Guillain-Barré syndrome. *Arch Neurol*. 1977;34:576–577.
70. Daube JR, Kelly JJ, Martin RA. Facial myokymia with polyradiculoneuropathy. *Neurology*. 1979;29:662–669.
71. Gutmann L. AAEM minimonograph #37: Facial and limb myokymia. *Muscle Nerve*. 1991;14:1043–1049.
72. Kennedy RH, Danielson MA, Mulder DW, Kurland LT. Guillain-Barré syndrome: a 42 year epidemiologic and clinical study. *Mayo Clin Proc*. 1978;53:93–99.
73. Andersson T, Siden A. A clinical study of the Guillain-Barré syndrome. *Acta Neurol Scand*. 1982;66:316–327.
74. Marshall J. The Landry-Guillain-Barré syndrome. *Brain*. 1963;86:55–66.
75. Wiederholt WC, Mulder DW, Lambert EH. The Landry-Guillain-Barré-Strohl syndrome or polyradiculoneuropathy: historical review, report on 97 patients, and present concepts. *Mayo Clin Proc*. 1964;39:427–451.
76. Ravn H. The Landry-Guillain-Barré syndrome. A survey and a clinical report of 127 cases. *Acta Neurol Scand*. 1967;43(suppl 30):1–64.
77. Loffel NB, Rossi LN, Mumenthaler M, Lutschg J, Ludin H-P. The Landry-Guillain-Barré syndrome. Complications, prognosis and natural history in 123 cases. *J Neurol Sci*. 1977;33:71–79.
78. Kaeser HE. Klinische und elektromyographische verlaufsuntersuchungen beim Guillain-Barré syndrom. *Schweiz Arch Neurol Neurochir Psychiat*. 1964;94:278–286.
79. Osler LD, Sidell AD. The Guillain-Barré syndrome. The need for exact diagnostic criteria. *N Engl J Med*. 1960;262:964–969.
80. Morley JB, Reynolds EH. Papilloedema and the Landry-Guillain-Barré syndrome. *Brain*. 1966;89:205–222.
81. Forster FM, Brown M, Merritt HH. Polyneuritis with facial diplegia: a clinical study. *N Engl J Med*. 1941;225:51–56.
82. Duvoisin RC. Polyneuritis: clinical review of 23 cases of Landry-Guillain-Barré syndrome. *US Armed Forces Med J*. 1960;11:1294–1306.
83. Pleasure DE, Lovelace RE, Duvoisin RC. The prognosis of acute polyradiculoneuritis. *Neurology*. 1968;18:1143–1148.
84. Raman PT, Taori GM. Prognostic significance of electrodiagnostic studies in the Guillain-Barré syndrome. *J Neurol Neurosurg Psychiatry*. 1976;39:163–170.
85. Miller RG, Peterson GW, Daube JR, Albers JW. Prognostic value of electrodiagnosis in Guillain-Barré syndrome. *Muscle Nerve*. 1988;11:769–774.
86. Winer JB, Greenwood RJ, Hughes RAC, Perkin GD, Healy MJR. Prognosis in Guillain-Barré syndrome. *Lancet*. 1985;1:1202–1203.
87. Peterman AF, Daly DD, Dion RF, Keith HM. Infectious neuronitis (Guillain-Barré syndrome) in children. *Neurology*. 1959;9:533–539.
88. Rantala H, Uhari M, Niemela M. Occurrence, clinical manifestations, and prognosis of Guillain-Barré syndrome. *Arch Dis Child*. 1991;66:706–709.
89. Bradshaw DY, Jones HR Jr. Guillain-Barré syndrome in children: clinical course, electrodiagnosis and prognosis. *Muscle Nerve*. 1992;15:500–506.
90. Berglund A. Polyradikulonevriter. *Nord Med*. 1954;52:1091–1095.
91. Cornblath DR, Mellits ED, Griffin JW, et al. Motor conduction studies in Guillain-Barré syndrome: description and prognostic value. *Ann Neurol*. 1988;23:354–359.
92. McKhann GM, Griffin JW, Cornblath DR, et al. Plasmapheresis and Guillain-Barré syndrome: analysis of prognostic factors and the effects of plasmapheresis. *Ann Neurol*. 1988;23:347–353.
93. Triggs WJ, Gominak SC, Cros DP, et al. Inexcitable motor nerves and low amplitude motor responses in the Guillain-Barré syndrome: distal conduction block or severe axonal degeneration? *Muscle Nerve*. 1991;14:892–893.

5

Treatment I: Supportive Care

Guillain-Barré syndrome (GBS) is a disease in which 85% of patients will make a complete functional recovery. It is therefore doubly imperative that any treatment adhere to one of the basic tenets of the Hippocratic principle, namely, "never do harm to anyone." Although some recently introduced treatments appear to accelerate the rate of recovery and may reduce the residual neurological deficit, the primary goal of treatment is still to provide supportive care during the acute illness so that the natural process of recovery by remyelination can occur.[1-3] Because of the substantial risks attendant on respiratory failure and autonomic instability, all patients with GBS, no matter how mild it may initially appear, should be admitted to a hospital with intensive care unit (ICU) facilities. It is impractical to expect all patients to be admitted to an ICU but anyone with declining pulmonary function or those with demonstrated autonomic instability, manifested as cardiac arrhythmias or unstable blood pressure, should be closely monitored in the intensive care setting.

Respiratory Care

Respiratory failure constituted the major cause of death in GBS until the acceleration of technology in the field of artificial ventilation.[4] These advances are largely responsible for the progressive decline in mortality during the 1950s and 1960s. In the early 1950s the mortality was approximately 15%,[5,6] but it was less than 5% after 1960.[7,8] In one study from the 1970s, mortality was 3.8% (3/79) during a 6-year period, even though 26% of the patients had disease of sufficient severity to necessitate treatment in an ICU and 16%

needed nasotracheal intubation.[9] In two recent multicenter studies of plasmapheresis, including both treated and untreated patients, there were only 7 deaths in 245 patients (2.9%)[10] and 14 deaths in 220 patients (6.4%).[11] At the Massachusetts General Hospital between 1962 and 1979 the overall mortality was 1.25% in all patients, 29% of whom required mechanical ventilation.[3] From the same institution, after 1980, Ropper and Kehne[12] reported a mortality rate of 3% in a select group of 38 severely involved patients who were sufficiently unstable to be admitted to the ICU; none of the patients requiring mechanical ventilation died. Today, deaths from respiratory failure alone should be rare, although some mortality from the respiratory complications of artificial ventilation and immobility remains inevitable, particularly in elderly patients.

Respiratory failure necessitating mechanical ventilation occurs in up to 25% of patients.[8,9,13,14] It is critically important to recognize that respiratory failure in GBS is not necessarily confined to those patients with severe appendicular paralysis. For example, respiratory failure has been described in patients with Miller-Fisher syndrome.[15,16] In addition, rapid deterioration over a few hours may occur in patients with seemingly trivial neuropathy when first seen. Therefore, all patients with GBS, regardless of severity, should be admitted to the hospital and closely monitored. They should be evaluated at the time of admission with pulmonary function tests. These provide essential information regarding the degree of covert deterioration of respiratory function and can also help to determine whether preexisting pulmonary disease is present. The latter, particularly chronic obstructive pulmonary disease, will increase the risk of developing respiratory failure as neuromuscular function deteriorates and may influence the management of patients as respiratory compromise supervenes. Although a wide variety of sophisticated and sensitive measures of pulmonary function is available, the best ones to use are those that are simple to administer and not unnecessarily tiring to the patient.[17] Tidal volume (TV) and respiratory rate (RR) provide useful information and have the advantage that they are highly reproducible in these weak and anxious patients, primarily because they require little patient cooperation. However, the vital capacity (VC) remains the gold standard and should be recorded regularly in all patients. It has the disadvantage that it requires full patient cooperation, which may be difficult in fatigued patients, and is therefore not so reproducible. In addition, if there is facial weakness, it may be difficult to achieve a complete seal around the mouthpiece; if there is palatal weakness there may be air loss through the nose, giving spurious results. If the ratio, TV/RR, falls below 10 or the VC falls below 15 ml/kg body weight, the patient should receive assisted ventilation.[3] If bulbar function is compromised or if the patient is becoming unduly fatigued, the threshold for intubation and assisted ventilation will be lower (VC 18 ml/kg). Baseline arterial blood gases should also be measured and repeated whenever there is any clinical suggestion of pulmonary compromise. Seemingly trivial hypoxemia may be a harbinger of overt respiratory failure and may exacerbate the risk for developing arrhythmias in those patients with autonomic instability. The chest radiograph should be examined for evidence of atelectasis and preexisting pulmonary disease.

Once patients have had these baseline parameters measured, they then need to be monitored closely for signs of impending respiratory failure. Although a fixed tachycardia is common in patients with GBS, an increasing heart rate, especially if accompanied by an increasing respiratory rate, is an important sign of deteriorating pulmonary function and has the practical advantage of being easy to monitor without unduly disturbing the patient. Excessive sweating may be an important clinical sign of increased respiratory effort and developing fatigue, although it may also be seen with autonomic instability related to the underlying neuropathy. The VC and TV/RR ratio should be recorded at least three times each day and more often if deterioration occurs.

Arterial blood gases should be measured at the first sign of deterioration of mechanical respiratory functions. The earliest change is mild hypoxemia with normal pco_2, secondary to shunting of venous blood through areas of microatelectasis.[18] Hypercarbia is a much later feature. It is important that endotracheal intubation and mechanical ventilation be started before the patient becomes exhausted and develops overt respiratory failure, manifested as hypercarbia and hypoxia. Sustained hypoxia, even when mild, may be complicated by sudden cardiac arrest, especially in those patients who may have autonomic instability. Fatigue of respiratory muscles is an important and underappreciated aspect of neuromuscular respiratory failure. The neural drive to respiratory muscles in an attempt to maintain a normal pco_2 can produce rapidly progressive muscle fatigue even without progression of the underlying neuromuscular disease.[19] Therefore, intubation should be carried out early, before fatigue becomes prominent and accelerated deterioration of respiratory function occurs. If endotracheal intubation is required for more than 5 to 7 days, tracheostomy probably should be performed to avoid the late complication of tracheal stenosis, although endotracheal intubation for much longer periods has been used without complication in both adults and children.[20,21]

The timing of weaning from mechanical ventilation requires considerable clinical judgment. Intermittent mandatory ventilation (IMV), in which the patient triggers the ventilator during attempted inspiration, should first be instituted. The IMV rate is then lowered to encourage patients to use their own muscles more. Careful monitoring of blood gases for signs of fatigue is important but fatigue is less of a problem during weaning since the neuropathy is steadily improving. Once the VC exceeds 15 ml/kg most patients can be weaned, although continued assisted ventilation during sleep may be necessary for a few days. Factors independent of the neuropathy, such as infection, anemia, or electrolyte disturbances, may interfere with weaning. In addition, patients with a prior history of pulmonary disease, particularly chronic bronchitis and emphysema, will be much more difficult to wean.

Management of Autonomic Instability

The severity of the autonomic neuropathy is usually proportional to the somatic neuropathy. However, as is the case with respiratory failure, autonomic instability is not confined to patients with severe paralysis. Several cases have been reported in which the presenting feature was autonomic failure with paralysis occurring later.[22–24] All patients with GBS should therefore be monitored closely for signs of autonomic instability.

Urinary retention is relatively common and intermittent catheterization may be necessary. Indwelling urinary catheters should be avoided because of the risk of developing nosocomial infection. Most patients will not need catheterization after the first few days of the illness, as long as they are able to communicate the need to void. Carbachol and other cholinergic drugs should be avoided since they may precipitate or exacerbate cardiac arrhythmias. Constipation is also common and is exacerbated by inactivity and the use of narcotics for pain. Ileus is a rare manifestation of the autonomic neuropathy. Constipation should be treated as conservatively as possible with stool softeners, bulk laxatives, or rectal suppositories. Avoidance of straining is important as it may cause or exacerbate hypotension and cardiac arrhythmias.

Persistent resting tachycardia is common but requires no active intervention. More serious arrhythmias, such as ventricular ectopy and atrioventricular conduction defects, are rare and should be treated with appropriate antiarrhythmic drugs or cardiac pacing. Prophylactic use of a demand pacemaker has been suggested for patients with bradycardia, even in the absence of atrioventricular conduction defects.[25–27]

Blood pressure may be low but is more often high and may vacillate widely over short intervals. Hypotension is best treated with volume expansion since pressor agents may be ineffective or may even precipitate dangerous hypertension. The autonomic neuropathy may result in denervation hypersensitivity, leading to this exaggerated response to vasopressors. Recognition of postural hypotension is important, particularly in ambulatory patients and when active rehabilitation starts. All patients should be checked for postural hypotension before active physical therapy begins. Elevated blood pressure is more common than overt hypotension, but is often transient. Hypertension usually does not need pharmacological treatment. Simple measures such as elevation of the head of the bed and allaying anxiety as much as possible may be all that is needed. If drugs are used, mild diuretics are usually safe but do increase renal sodium loss in patients who are already prone to hyponatremia. Rarely, if hypertension is severe and sustained, particularly in the elderly or those with overt ischemic heart disease, more aggressive treatment may be needed. Short-acting intravenous agents like sodium nitroprusside have the advantage that their action can be terminated rapidly if hypotension occurs. Hypertension may be related to increased renin secretion and therefore may be particularly responsive to beta-adrenergic blocking drugs such as propanolol. It has been suggested that alpha-adrenergic blockers should be given concomitantly since propranolol may increase the vasopressor response to increased levels of circulating catecholamines in GBS.

Management of Bulbar Palsy

The frequent combination of bulbar weakness with respiratory compromise is doubly dangerous and meticulous attention to secretions is critical. Frequent suctioning of secretions from the posterior pharynx is often necessary; occasionally endotracheal intubation or even tracheostomy is indicated to prevent aspiration in patients whose degree of respiratory compromise would not otherwise require ventilatory support. Anticholinergic drugs should not be used to reduce the production of secretions as they may cause or exacerbate autonomic instability. Stimulation of the nasopharynx or the more distal airways during suctioning and endotracheal intubation may also induce arrhythmias, but the benefit far outweighs the risk. Nonetheless, suctioning should be done as gently as possible. Bulbar palsy may also necessitate nasogastric intubation for feeding, which is preferable to intravenous hyperalimentation. If swallowing difficulties are prolonged over weeks, gastrostomy should be considered.

Treatment of the Complications of Respiratory Failure and Bulbar Paralysis

The two pulmonary complications that play a major role in the morbidity and mortality of GBS are bronchopneumonia and pulmonary embolism.[28,29]

Bronchopneumonia and Upper Airway Infection

Bronchopneumonia results from secondary infection of areas of atelactasis related to hypoventilation, aggravated by aspiration of secretions in patients with bulbar involvement. Occasionally, an antecedent pulmonary infection that may have triggered the GBS may persist until the onset of weakness and increase the risk of bronchopneumonia. Preexisting chronic bronchitis and other pulmonary diseases also increase this risk. Atelectasis may be prevented or reduced by vigorous respiratory therapy, which should be given at least daily in patients with declining respiratory status and usually more often. Meticulous pulmonary toilet will reduce the degree of aspiration and careful attention to hydration makes the removal of secretions easier. The use of prophylactic antibiotics for atelectasis alone is not indicated because of the risk of developing more serious, hospital-acquired infections. However, early detection of pneumonia through monitoring the temperature, examining the sputum and obtaining regular chest radiographs will allow for early antibiotic treatment of pneumonia if it does develop. The choice of antibiotic should be predicated on the results of sputum culture and should have a broad spectrum of activity.

Upper respiratory tract infection may also occur. Tracheitis is a particular problem in intubated patients. Fever and purulent sputum in the absence of chest radiograph infiltrates should raise this suspicion. Sinusitis and otitis also occasionally occur in intubated patients, possibly related to impairment of drainage due to the endotracheal tube.

Deep Venous Thrombosis and Pulmonary Embolism

Deep venous thrombosis with pulmonary embolism is common in patients whose weakness is sufficient to confine them to bed. In one study, one-third of patients developed pulmonary embolism.[29] Even weak patients should be ambulated if possible and should be consistently reminded to move if bedfast. However, ambulation of patients with muscular weakness and autonomic instability may produce postural hypotension and cardiac arrhythmias. Severely paralyzed patients should be passively moved as much as is feasible. Prophylactic, low dose, subcutaneous heparin (5000 units twice daily) should be given to patients confined to bed. Pulmonary embolism may be difficult to recognize as the characteristic abnormalities on chest radiographs, arterial blood gases, and even the nuclide ventilation-perfusion scan may be mimicked by the atelectasis alone, associated with arteriovenous shunting. If pulmonary embolism does occur, the patient should be evaluated and treated in the usual fashion, without specific regard to the GBS.

Prevention and Management of Infection

In addition to pulmonary infection discussed above, urinary tract infection is common in patients with GBS, particularly in patients in the ICU. This tendency is exacerbated by the frequent parasympathetic neuropathy resulting in increased urinary residual or even overt retention. About 20% of GBS patients will develop urinary infection requiring antibiotics.[3] Colonization of the urine with nosocomial organisms is almost inevitable with indwelling catheters for 5 or more days, but only patients with significant pyuria (>10 white blood cells per high power field) or evidence of systemic sepsis should be treated with systemic antibiotics. The urine should be checked microscopically at least twice weekly and cultured weekly. Enterococcal infection is particularly common. Choice of antibiotic depends on the sensitivity of the organism but high dose ampicillin is usually effective, even when sensitivity is not high.

Management of Fluid Balance and Nutrition

A careful record of fluid balance should be kept for all patients with respiratory failure or significant swallowing difficulties. Insensible fluid losses need to be replaced but overhydration should be avoided. Insensible loss will be increased by fever. Inappropriate secretion of antidiuretic hormone occasionally complicates GBS and hyponatremia may result, especially in mechanically ventilated patients. Pure dextrose intravenous solutions should be avoided to prevent exacerbation of hyponatremia; normal saline with 0.5% to 1.0% dextrose should be used. Potassium loss is increased in acute illness and potassium supplementation (100 mmol daily) should be given.

The stress of an acute illness increases caloric expenditure but paralysis reduces the requirement for calories. In general, feeding of patients unable to swallow is not necessary for the first week. Thereafter, undernutrition may lead to hypoalbuminemia and may increase the risk of skin breakdown in these immobile patients. Nasogastric intubation for feeding is preferable to intravenous hyperalimentation, but wide-bore tubes should be avoided as they may cause gastric erosion and increase the risk of regurgitation and aspiration. Immobile patients require about 1500 to 2000 calories a day. Commercially available high-calorie formulas are available but should be used in a diluted form at first to avoid diarrhea. Frequent small-volume feedings (approximately 50 ml every 2 hr) may be inconvenient but are better tolerated than larger volumes. Sepsis increases caloric requirements to 2500 to 3000 calories daily and may necessitate hyperalimentation. The stress of illness and the inevitable frequent phlebotomy often lead to anemia. Iron replacement should be used if tolerated, but it frequently causes nausea or intolerance of nasogastric feedings. If the hematocrit falls below 28% to 30% transfusion may be necessary.

Care of the Immobile Patient

The major complications of immobility in patients with more severe GBS are contractures, decubitous ulcers, and deep venous thrombosis. Early involvement of physical therapists in the management of patients with GBS is important. Frequent turning of the patient will minimize the risk of developing decubiti and deep venous thrombosis but may cause significant discomfort to the patient, particularly early when pain may be severe. Use of analgesics before physical therapy is often helpful. A water or air mattress should be used to minimize skin breakdown. Paralyzed joints should be put through a full passive range of movement at least daily to prevent contractures. A board at the foot of the bed or molded ankle–foot orthoses may help in preventing foot drop and Achilles tendon contracture, and wrist splints may also be helpful. As soon as the risk of autonomic instability and respiratory compromise has passed, a program of more active rehabilitation should be instituted.

Treatment of Pain

Pain is a common symptom in GBS, occurring in 50% or more of patients and is often severe enough to warrant treatment.[30] It is particularly important to inquire specifically about pain in patients who are having difficulty communicating because of endotracheal intubation. Pain occurring early may be due to nerve or muscle edema and inflammation and may respond dramatically to plasmapheresis or corticosteroids. Later, distal dysesthetic pain with cutaneous hyperpathia may develop, presumably reflecting inflammatory injury to nociceptive afferent fibers. Symptomatic treatment of pain with simple analgesics such as aspirin or acetaminophen may be sufficient, but occasionally it is severe enough to warrant the use of narcotics. A few cases have been described with intractable pain, despite parenteral narcotics and a variety of other pharmacological agents, who responded dramatically to epidural opioids.[31,32] Quinine sulfate may also produce relief.[33] Other pharmacological agents that may be beneficial in pain management, such as tricyclic antidepressants, tranquilizers, anticonvulsants, benzodiazepines, and others, should be used with caution during the active phase of the illness because of their propensity to cause or exacerbate hypotension, cardiac arrhythmias, and respiratory depression. However, they have been used safely and with good effect.[34] Transcutaneous nerve stimulation may also help.[35] Hyperpathia and dysesthesiae may respond to topical capsaicin.[36] We have found that mexiletine (150–250 mg three times daily), a cardiac antiarrhythmic drug, is sometimes strikingly effective in the treatment of the later dysesthetic pain but it should be avoided in patients with autonomic instability because of its occasional tendency to exacerbate arrhythmias.

Emotional Support of the Patient and Family

Although GBS carries an excellent prognosis for complete functional recovery with time, patients and their families are invariably extremely anxious, particularly during the phase of the illness when deterioration is occurring.[37] Endotracheal intubation with confinement to an ICU, bulbar paralysis, and severe peripheral weakness all induce a profound feeling of helplessness and fear of death. It is hard to convince a patient that prognosis is good, when they see that each day appears worse than the one before. Nonetheless, it is important to emphasize the usual good outcome in all contacts with the patient and relatives. Contact with support groups, comprising recovered patients and their families, may be particularly helpful in this respect. It is equally important to set up methods for communication for all patients who are intubated so that they can apprise staff and family of their needs.

Summary

The best quality supportive care remains the cornerstone of the treatment of GBS despite recent advances in treating the disease itself. Meticulous attention must be paid to all GBS patients so that complications can be anticipated and prevented if possible, or at least recognized early so that appropriate treatment can be administered.

References

1. Hughes RAC, Kadlubowski M, Hufschmidt A. Treatment of acute inflammatory polyneuropathy. *Ann Neurol.* 1981;9(suppl):125–133.
2. Pollard JD. A critical review of therapies in acute and chronic inflammatory demyelinating polyneuropathies. *Muscle Nerve.* 1987;10:214–221.
3. Ropper AH, Shahani BT. Diagnosis and management of acute areflexic paralysis with emphasis on the Guillain-Barré syndrome. In: Asbury AK, Gilliatt RW, eds. *Peripheral nerve disorders.* London: Butterworths; 1984:21–45.
4. Hewer RL, Hilton PJ, Crampton-Smith A, Spalding JMK. Acute polyneuritis requiring artificial respiration. *Q J Med.* 1968;33:479–491.
5. Berglund A. Polyradikulonevriter. *Nord Med.* 1954;52:1091–1095.
6. Ravn H. The Landry-Guillain-Barré syndrome. A survey and a clinical report of 127 cases. *Acta Neurol Scand.* 1967;43(suppl 30):1–64.
7. Petlund CF. Polyradiculitis Guillain-Barré, et 10-ars-materiale. (Review of 10 years LGBS cases). *T Norske Laegeforen.* 1962;82:1139–1141.
8. Wiederholt CW, Mulder DW, Lambert EH. The Landry-Guillain-Barré-Strohl syndrome or polyradiculoneuropathy: historical review, report on 97 patients and present concepts. *Mayo Clin Proc.* 1964;39:427–451.
9. Gracey DR, McMichan JC, Divertie MB, Howard FM. Respiratory failure in Guillain-Barré syndrome. A 6-year experience. *Mayo Clin Proc.* 1982;57:742–746.
10. The Guillain-Barré Syndrome Study Group. Plasmapheresis and acute Guillain-Barré syndrome. *Neurology.* 1985;35:1096–1104.
11. French Cooperative Group on Plasma Exchange in Guillain-Barré Syndrome. Efficiency of plasma exchange in Guillain-Barré syndrome: role of replacement fluids. *Ann Neurol.* 1987; 22:753–761.
12. Ropper AH, Kehne SM. Guillain-Barré syndrome: management of respiratory failure. *Neurology.* 1985;35:1662–1665.
13. Dowling PC, Menonna JP, Cook SD. Guillain-Barré syndrome in Greater New York, New Jersey. *JAMA.* 1977;238:317–318.
14. Loffel NB, Rossi LN, Mumenthaler M, Lutschg J, Ludin HP. The Landry-Guillain-Barré syndrome—complications, prognosis and natural history in 123 cases. *J Neurol Sci.* 1977; 33:71–79.
15. Blau I, Casson I, Lieberman A, Weiss E. The not so benign Miller Fisher syndrome. *Arch Neurol.* 1980;37:384–385.
16. Littlewood R, Bajada S. Successful plasmapheresis in the Miller-Fisher syndrome. *Br Med J.* 1981;282:778–780.
17. Pontoppidan H, Geffin B, Lowenstein E. Acute respiratory failure in the adult. *N Engl J Med.* 1972;287:743–752.
18. Ringel SP, Carroll JE. Respiratory complications of neuromuscular disease. In: Weiner WJ, ed. *Respiratory dysfunction in neurologic disease.* Mt Kisco: Futura Publishing; 1980:113–115.
19. Roussos C, Macklem PT. The respiratory muscles. *N Engl J Med.* 1982;307:786–797.
20. Newsum JK, Smith RM, Crocker D. Intubation for respiratory failure in the Guillain-Barré syndrome. *JAMA.* 1979;242:1650–1651.
21. Stauffer JL, Olson DE, Petty TL. Complications and consequences of endotracheal intubation and tracheotomy. A prospective study of 150 critically ill adult patients. *Am J Med.* 1981; 70:65–76.

22. Birchfield RI, Shaw C-M. Postural hypotension in the Guillain-Barré syndrome. *Arch Neurol.* 1964;10:149–157.
23. Hodson AK, Hurwitz BJ, Albrecht R. Dysautonomia in Guillain-Barré syndrome with dorsal root ganglioneuropathy, Wallerian degeneration and fatal myocarditis. *Ann Neurol.* 1984; 15:88–95.
24. Wani BA, Misra M, Shah M, Mufti S. Acute inflammatory demyelinating polyradiculo-neuropathy presenting as complete heart block and Stoke-Adam attacks. *Postgrad Med J.* 1989;65:103–104.
25. Emmons PR, Blume WT, DuShane JW. Cardiac monitoring and demand pacemaker in Guillain-Barré syndrome. *Arch Neurol.* 1975;32:59–61.
26. Favre H, Foex P, Guggisberg M. Use of demand pacemaker in a case of Guillain-Barré syndrome. *Lancet.* 1970;1:1062–1063.
27. Greenland P, Griggs RC. Arrhythmic complications in the Guillain-Barré syndrome. *Arch Intern Med.* 1980;140:1053–1055.
28. Haymaker W, Kernohan JW. Landry-Guillain-Barré syndrome: clinicopathological report of 50 fatal cases and a critique of the literature. *Medicine (Baltimore).* 1949;28:59–141.
29. Raman TK, Blake JA, Harris TM. Pulmonary embolism in Landry-Guillain-Strohl syndrome. *Chest.* 1971;60:555–557.
30. Ropper AH, Shahani BT. Pain in the Guillain-Barré syndrome. *Arch Neurol.* 1984;41:511–514.
31. Connelly M, Shagrin J, Warfield C. Epidural opioids for the management of pain in a patient with the Guillain-Barré syndrome. *Anesthesiology.* 1990;72:381–383.
32. Rosenfield B, Burel C, Hanley D. Epidural morphine treatment of pain in Guillain-Barré syndrome. *Arch Neurol.* 1986;43:1194–1196.
33. Nixon RA. Quinine sulfate for pain in the Guillain-Barré syndrome. *Ann Neurol.* 1978;4: 386–387.
34. Winspur I. Tegretol for pain in the Guillain-Barré syndrome. *Lancet.* 1970;637:85.
35. McCarthy JA, Zigensfus RW. Transcutaneous nerve stimulation: an adjunct in the pain management of Guillain-Barré syndrome. *Phys Ther.* 1978;58:23–24.
36. Morgenlander JC, Hurwitz BJ, Massey EW. Capsaicin for the treatment of pain in Guillain-Barré syndrome. *Ann Neurol.* 1990;28:199.
37. Shearn MA, Shearn L. A personal experience with Guillain-Barré syndrome: are the psychologic needs of patients and family being met? *South Med J.* 1986;79:800–803.

6

Treatment II: Immunotherapy of Guillain-Barré Syndrome

The evidence that Guillain-Barré syndrome (GBS) is an autoimmune disease is circumstantial but overwhelming. Therefore, attempts to attenuate the severity of the disease and accelerate remission have concentrated on manipulation of the immune system. Until recently, there was considerable controversy concerning the role of immune manipulation in GBS, but recent controlled trials have established a role for plasmapheresis and for high-dose intravenous immunoglobulin. The use of corticosteroids and other immunosuppressives is unjustified given the lack of evidence of efficacy and the not insubstantial risk.

Plasmapheresis

A plethora of anecdotal reports, attesting to the effectiveness of plasmapheresis in GBS, first appeared between 1978 and 1980 and continued to proliferate in the early 1980s.[1-5] Plasmapheresis was even used in a patient with Miller-Fisher syndrome.[6] Most of the reports were euphoric, but occasionally caution was voiced. For example, neither of the two GBS patients treated by Cook et al.[7] improved with plasmapheresis, although they noted that neither had further progression of symptoms after the first treatment.

Three of these early studies were controlled by randomization of patients but involved small patient numbers. Greenwood and associates,[8] in a study of 30 patients randomly allocated to plasmapheresis or no treatment, were unable to demonstrate a significant benefit to the treated patients and concluded that the treatment was not justified. Similarly, Murray and associates[9] compared the effects of plasmapheresis in seven patients with six who received no treatment other than an oral placebo and found no clinical or electrophysiological differences between the two groups at 3 months. However, Osterman and associates[10] compared 18 treated patients with 20 controls and found that the treated patients improved more rapidly. Significant differences were apparent as early as 1 month but were greater by 2 months. An important difference between this and previous studies was that patients were admitted to treatment much earlier. Later, Bezwoda and associates[11] compared the outcome in 15 patients treated with plasmapheresis with a group retrospectively matched for disease severity. They also found a significant benefit with respect to duration of weakness and length of hospitalization. Mendell and coworkers,[12] in a study of 25 patients, were unable to demonstrate a benefit. In their study, patients were treated with both plasmapheresis and prednisone and they postulate that the failure may have reflected an adverse effect of the steroids.

The rationale for the use of plasmapheresis is easy to understand. Circulating antibodies to peripheral nerve have often been demonstrated in GBS patients, although their significance in the pathogenesis of the disease or the production of symptoms remains controversial. However, in 1971 it was demonstrated that sera from patients with GBS were able to produce primary demyelination, without axonal degeneration, in myelinated peripheral nerves in tissue culture.[13] The reaction was complement dependent and the ability to demyelinate resided in both the 7S and 19S gammaglobulin fractions. The demyelinating factors in serum were not specific for GBS but were also seen in a variety of other central and peripheral nervous system disorders, not necessarily demyelinating in nature. However, demyelination was much more frequent and severe with serum from patients with GBS. Furthermore, in sera from GBS patients, demyelination was more frequent and severe when symptoms were of less than 3 weeks' duration, suggesting a pathogenetic role of these antibodies in the demyelination of GBS. Subsequently, several investigators demonstrated that sera from patients with GBS produced demyelination *in vivo*, when introduced directly into the endoneurial compartment, thus circumventing the perineurial and endothelial barriers.[14–18] Not everyone was able to confirm these results. For example, Low and associates[19] found no difference in the degree of demyelination between GBS and control sera. In the study of Saida and associates,[17] all sera were obtained within the first 3 weeks of onset of symptoms and were stored for varying lengths of time. They found a significant correlation between disease severity and extent of demyelination but no correlation between duration of disease or length of storage. By contrast, Feasby et al.[15] and Harrison et al.[16] collected sera from a few days to many months after the onset of symptoms and found that over these periods of time the demyelinating activity of the sera declined significantly. Although in each of these *in vivo* studies sera from both normal controls and patients with a variety of other neurological disorders also produced demyelination, GBS sera were much more potent. Subsequently, Heininger et al.[20] were able to transfer demyelination passively from a patient with the chronic form of inflammatory demyelinating neuropathy to monkeys by systemically injecting multiple doses of IgG, indicating that the demyelinating factor was an immunoglobulin. Their patient had been particularly responsive to plasmapheresis. Koski et al.[21] found anti-peripheral nerve myelin antibodies in all GBS patients tested and there was a close correlation between the antibody titer and the clinical course of the disease. Metral et al.[22] found that the serum factor that produced conduction block in recipient animals after intraneural injection diminished in parallel with clinical improvement and that it was still present at 1 year only in those patients with significant motor sequelae. The nature of the circulating demyelinating factor remains obscure. Interest focused on antibodies to galactocerebroside because these had been shown previously to produce demyelination when injected intraneurally into the sciatic nerve. However, antigalactocerebroside antibodies could not be found in the serum or cerebrospinal fluid (CSF) of patients with GBS.[23] Antibodies to a variety of gangliosides have been demonstrated in GBS patients but it has not been shown whether they possess demyelinating activity.[24] These *in vitro* and *in vivo* studies provide strong evidence that circulating antibodies play a role in the pathogenesis of demyelination in GBS and that the concentration of these antibodies, or at least the demyelinating activity of the sera, is highest in those patients with the most severe paralysis and earliest in the course of the disease.

Because of the strong rationale for the use of plasmapheresis in GBS and the controversy generated by the several small studies and anecdotal reports, a multicenter, randomized trial of plasmapheresis was started in North America in 1980 and the results were reported in 1985.[25] One hundred twenty-two patients were treated with plasmapheresis and 123 received conventional, supportive treatment. To be eligible for admission to the study, the patients had to have disease of sufficient severity to prevent walking. Treatment consisted of exchanging 200 to 250 ml of plasma/kg body weight over 7 to 14 days. Replacement was with a variety of fluids including plasmanate, albumen, and pooled plasma. Patients were treated with both continuous and intermittent flow machines. There was no difference between the two groups in terms of mortality or relapses of the GBS. However, in almost all other respects, the treated patients fared better. Specifically, patients improved more rapidly, required less ventilator assistance, spent less time in intensive care units, and less overall time in the hospital. This benefit was seen at 4 weeks and at 6 months after the onset of symptoms. Consistent with the previously reported findings of highest demyelinating activity in sera taken during the early days of the illness, plasmapheresis was most beneficial when started early, within a week of the onset of symptoms. If treatment was started more than 2 weeks after onset of symptoms there was no demonstrable benefit. Subsequent data analysis indicated that patients treated with continuous flow machines fared better than those on intermittent flow.[26] Although patients with electrophysiological evidence of associated axonal degeneration consistently fared worse, plasmapheresis also improves the prognosis in this subgroup of patients.[27]

This trial established a high probability that plasmapheresis was an effective and safe method for treating patients with GBS and has formed the basis for therapeutic decisions since its publication. A similarly designed French multicenter trial published in 1987 also demonstrated a significant benefit and found, in addition, that the replacement fluid did not influence outcome.[28] Dyck and Kurtzke[29] suggested that this might have influenced the outcome in some cases in the North American trial, since intravenous hyperimmuneglobulin has been shown to affect beneficially the outcome of chronic inflammatory demyelinating neuropathy. Curiously, a small, prospective, randomized study of the effect of plasmapheresis reported from Finland found that quantitative measures of muscle strength improved more in treated patients but the benefits of shortened hospital and intensive care unit (ICU) stays were not found.[30]

In randomized trials in Sweden,[10] North America,[25] and France,[28] treated patients all fell into the severe category. The first two intentionally restricted entry on the basis of severity and in the French study, although no such restrictions were imposed, 95% of patients had severe disease. There are no data on the safety and efficacy of plasmapheresis in mild GBS, although it is most likely to be of equal or greater benefit. However, its cost effectiveness will be considerably reduced since many patients with mild disease are destined to remain mild and would not require any treatment. De Silva et al.[31] studied the effect of a highly cost effective method of plasma exchange, applicable for use in developing countries or any center where more sophisticated technology is unavailable. They removed 0.5 liters of blood and replaced it with 0.25 liters of fresh frozen plasma. They then centrifuged the patient's blood, discarded the plasma, and returned the red blood cells. The procedure was done twice daily for 7 to 13 days on six patients, five of whom improved rapidly. Although this study was not controlled, it does suggest that the technique is effective and may have an important role in poorer areas of the world.

Few children were included in either of the major controlled studies. In the French study, patients had to be at least 16 years of age and in the North American study, at least 12. In the latter it is unclear how many children were treated. However, plasmapheresis has been found to be both safe and effective in children, even as young as 11 months. In one study, Epstein and Sladky compared 9 children who had been treated with plasmapheresis with 14 who received no specific treatment.[32] The groups were similar with respect to age, severity of disease, and duration of disease. Treated children returned to independent ambulation in 24 days compared to 60 days for untreated children. Others have also confirmed the safety of plasmapheresis in children with GBS and have suggested that it is effective.[33–35] However, none of these studies of plasmapheresis in childhood GBS has been controlled and the results of the uncontrolled studies have been criticized.[36,37] It therefore seems prudent to withhold plasmapheresis in children unless there is severe disease.

Although there is remarkable unanimity regarding the efficacy of plasma-pheresis with regard to accelerating recovery, there are few data on its ability to affect the progressively deteriorating phase of the disease. However, the French cooperative study suggests that early treatment does limit progression if started early enough. This provides an extra incentive to begin treatment early.

These studies have raised a therapeutic dilemma. To have maximum efficacy, treatment should be started as soon as possible. However, many patients are only mildly affected early in the course of the disease and consequently may not need treatment. Attempts to identify patients prospectively who are likely to need plasmapheresis have so far been unsuccessful. Osterman et al.[38] found that patients with complement fixing antibodies had more severe disease but there was no correlation between these, or other, antibodies and the subsequent course of the disease. At present it seems advisable to withhold treatment from mildly affected individuals but to follow them closely and begin treatment as soon as they are no longer able to walk or if significant respiratory or bulbar involvement supervenes. If progression is hyperacute treatment should be started earlier. In addition, when the antecedent event is of a type known to be associated with severe disease (such as with rabies vaccination and possibly surgery) and when there is a short duration between antecedent event and the onset of neurological symptoms (which also may anticipate severe disease), the threshold for beginning plasmapheresis should be lower.

Although plasmapheresis is usually a safe procedure and neither of the major studies reported significant adverse effects of the treatment, it should not be used in a cavalier fashion. In the North American trial 12 patients (10%) were withdrawn either by themselves or by their treating physicians for a variety of reasons. A similar percentage were withdrawn from the French trial. Hypotension, cardiac arrhythmias, sepsis, and both thrombotic and hemorrhagic complications of plasmapheresis have been reported. Nonetheless, in neither of these large trials was there any significant adverse outcome related to treatment except for a slight increase in sepsis in the French trial. However, particular care should be taken in patients with significant autonomic instability and the occasional complications argue even more persuasively for avoiding plasmapheresis in mildly affected patients.

It has also been suggested that plasmapheresis increases the relapse rate. Relapse rate was identical in the two groups in the North American study. In the French study, there were six relapses in the treated group compared with only one in the untreated group, but this difference was not statistically significant. However, Osterman et al.[39,40] and Ropper et al.[41] both report increased relapse rates in treated patients and our own experience confirms this impression. Rudnicki et al. reported some patients in whom relapse following plasmapheresis was accompanied by a rebound increase in anti-peripheral nerve myelin antibody, supporting the concept that these antibodies are important in the pathogenesis of demyelination.[42] The relapses are usually mild and respond to retreatment. It is important that patients be followed closely after treatment is completed to ensure that, if relapse does occur, it can be treated appropriately.

Corticosteroids

The first report of the use of corticosteroids in a predominantly motor neuropathy, which was probably GBS, largely reflects current opinion. In their review of the use of steroids in several neurological disorders, Shy and McEarchern[43] found no response in the three patients with acute neuropathy. Similarly, Plum,[44] in reviewing 3 years of experience with corticosteroids in GBS, concluded that there were occasional responses to steroids but that they were unpredictable and possibly coincidental. However, most of the early reports in the 1950s and 1960s, based entirely on anecdotal and retrospective experiences, were largely euphoric.[45,46] Several extensive studies in the 1960s, involving more than 150 cases, concluded that steroids arrested the progress of the disease, that patients improved more rapidly, and that mortality was reduced.[45–49] In 1963, Heller and DeJong reviewed the literature and added 18 cases of their own, concluding that the results suggested a "favorable response to hormone treatment in most patients who received it."[45] In 1968, Frick and Angstwurm compared the results from 37 patients treated with 30 to 50 mg of prednisolone daily with 29 untreated patients.[47] Although they report that treated patients improved more quickly, it is noteworthy that the hospital stay was longer, perhaps as a result of steroid-related complications. In another retrospective study from the Mayo Clinic, Wiederholt et al.[49] compared 22 patients treated with steroids with 68 patients who did not receive steroids. They also found that in steroid-treated patients the time to onset of improvement was more rapid but there was no significant effect on the overall duration of the neurological deficit.

Considering the widespread use of corticosteroids for the treatment of GBS over four decades and its continued use today, there has been a remarkable paucity of controlled trials of their efficacy. In 1976, Swick and McQuillen[50] carried out the first prospective, double-blind, placebo-controlled trial of adrenocorticotrophic hormone (ACTH). The nine treated patients received 100 units ACTH intramuscularly daily for 10 days whereas the controls were injected with the diluent. In addition, another eight patients who required ventilator assistance or had severe cranial nerve involvement were excluded from randomization but were given either ACTH or oral corticosteroids. Their outcome was compared with 14 similarly severe patients who had been seen previously and who had received no steroids. In both the randomized patients and the group as a whole, the time to onset of recovery occurred earlier in treated patients. However, steroids did not affect the total duration of the illness or alter the severity of the paralysis. Thus, the effects of steroids were minimal and the benefit probably insufficient to justify recommendation of their widespread use. In addition, 11 of the 16 randomized patients and 24 of the entire group were children (under 15 years of age) and extrapolation of results from such a nonrepresentative group to the general GBS population is unjustified. The results of a multicenter controlled trial in 40 patients was reported in 1978[51] that was not double-blind or placebo-controlled, although all clinical assessments were carried out by a neurologist who was unaware of the treatment status of the patients. Patients were randomly allocated to oral prednisolone (60 mg daily for 1 week and a tapering dose for a second week) or no steroid treatment. In this study, there was no benefit in terms of neurological disability in patients evaluated at 1, 3, and 12 months from the onset of paralysis. In fact, patients who received steroids uniformly fared worse than controls and the difference was significant 3 months into the illness. Furthermore, these investigators found that 3 of 21 patients receiving steroids relapsed after treatment was stopped compared with none of 19 controls. Others have also suggested that the relapse may be higher in patients receiving steroids.[46,48] Although the controlled studies of corticosteroids in GBS have yielded negative or unimpressively positive results, the total number of patients was small and the statistical power of the results low, making the possibility of a Type II (false negative) error large.

There have been anecdotal reports of response to high dose intravenous corticosteroids when oral dosage has failed. In one patient,[52] high dose oral prednisolone failed to arrest deterioration but intravenous (IV) injection of the same dose produced a prompt improvement. Change from IV to oral treatment on two subsequent occasions resulted in a rapid relapse followed by equally rapid improvement when IV treatment was reinstituted. Dowling et al.[53] report dramatic improvement in three of five GBS patients within hours of the administration of high dose IV prednisolone (500 mg daily). Encouraged by these observations, Haab et al.[54] administered 500 or 1000 mg of methylprednisolone intravenously to 11 GBS patients in an unblinded fashion and were encouraged by the results. They suggest that the dose should be given four times daily to avoid fluctuation in the plasma concentration.

Although the occasional dramatic response to steroids in some cases cannot be ignored, there is no conclusive evidence of overall benefit and, to date, there is no way of predicting those patients who may respond. Given the suggestion that treated patients may fare worse and the undoubted risks of high dose steroids, it seems prudent to advise that steroids not be used until more convincing evidence of benefit is available. Perhaps spurred on by these uncontrolled reports of dramatic improvement with high dose intravenous steroids, a study of the effects of methylprednisolone in GBS was started in

1988 and the early results were recently reported.[55] Two hundred forty-two patients were randomly and blindly allocated to treatment with IV methylprednisolone (500 mg daily for 5 days) or with placebo. This preliminary communication reported on the results of all patients who had reached 4 weeks after trial entry. Although the steroid-treated patients fared slightly better in terms of degree and rapidity of improvement, the advantage was trivial and entirely insignificant.

In summary, there is no evidence to support the notion that steroids are effective in the treatment of GBS, despite the overwhelming evidence that it is an autoimmune disease and that other forms of immune manipulation are effective. Furthermore, there have been several reports of GBS developing during treatment with steroids,[56–58] including a patient receiving high dose methylprednisolone.[59] Continuation of the common practice of using steroids cannot, therefore, be recommended.

Other Immunosuppressive Treatment

Cytotoxic Drugs

A variety of other immunosuppressive drugs has been advocated for the treatment of GBS. The rationale for such therapy is based on observations that these drugs may prevent the development of experimental allergic neuritis (EAN) in animals when administered at the same time as the antigen and can significantly reduce the severity of the neuropathy when given at the time of onset of the clinical syndrome.[60,61] Since there is a wealth of evidence to indicate that EAN is a reasonable model of GBS, it was reasoned that the course of GBS should be significantly modified by the same drugs. The successful use of 6-mercaptopurine (6-MP) in a single patient purported to have GBS was first reported in 1965.[62] However, the case report clearly identifies the patient as having progression over almost a year, clearly not consistent with GBS. A later report also noted the efficacy of azathioprine but again the patient had a prolonged course inconsistent with GBS.[63] Another report by Colin-Jones and Heathfield also describes a case of relapsing neuropathy successfully treated with 6-MP.[64] A number of subsequent individual case reports attested to the efficacy of 6-MP and azathioprine in subacute and relapsing neuropathies. In 1970, Yuill et al.[65] described five patients with acute neuropathy who had failed to respond to ACTH but responded after the administration of azathioprine. Rosen and Vastola[66] used high dose IV cyclophosphamide to treat 15 patients with neuropathy, 14 of whom probably had GBS. Some patients were treated more than once. Progression of the disease stopped in association with 21 courses of treatment and improvement was noted in 19. However, the ultimate degree of recovery was not different from what was expected in untreated patients. They describe reversible alopecia and nausea and vomiting as the only complications.

However, there were three deaths, which is dramatically higher than would be expected with supportive care alone. Although no controlled studies have been done, it is clear from the fragmentary literature that there is no justification for the use of these potentially dangerous drugs for the treatment of a disease in which most patients will recover and for which satisfactory, better tolerated, and infinitely safer alternatives are available.

Intravenous Immunoglobulin

Intravenous infusion of plasma or human immunoglobulin (IVIG) has been reported to produce dramatic improvement in patients with a variety of neurological and nonneurological autoimmune disorders,[67–69] including chronic inflammatory demyelinating neuropathy.[70,71] As with steroids and the early reports on plasmapheresis, most of the reports suffer from a lack of rigorous scientific method but are persuasive nonetheless. Several patients had been unresponsive to high dose steroids, plasmapheresis, and other immunosuppressives and yet have improved with IVIG. None of the treated patients suffered adverse effects of sufficient magnitude to warrant cessation of therapy. Early reports of the use of IVIG in the treatment of GBS are similarly tantalizing and are reminiscent of the early reports of the efficacy of plasmapheresis. Kleyweg et al.[72] report on their experience with IVIG treatment (0.4 g/kg/day for 4 days) in eight patients who seemed either to stop progressing or started to improve coincidental with the institution of treatment. Mauro[73] reported a single patient with GBS who had not improved with plasmapheresis but improved rapidly after high dose IVIG, administered at a dose of 0.4 g/kg/day for 3 days and then followed by a maintenance schedule of 0.4 g/kg every 15 days until sustained improvement was seen. IVIG has also been safely and successfully administered to children with GBS. Shahar et al.[74,75] and Lavenstein et al.[76] administered IVIG as the primary treatment of six children and noted dramatic improvement coincident with treatment. Jackson and Donnelly[77] treated two children who had not responded to plasmapheresis or in whom it could not be continued and also noted rapid improvement that they felt was not consistent with the natural history of the disease. Other, published[78] and unpublished, anecdotal reports of its efficacy abound.

These initial promising results have been confirmed in a prospective, randomized trial recently completed in the Netherlands[79] in which IVIG was compared with plasmapheresis. In this study, the patients treated with IVIG fared better in almost all respects. The time to recovery of locomotion was 14 days less for IVIG treated patients and the period of intubation was 7 days less. Patients were entered into the trial early, a mean of less than 6 days after the onset of symptoms and this enabled the effect of treatment on the progression of disease to be studied better. Almost twice as many patients required assisted ventilation in the plasmapheresis group, indicating a major benefit of IVIG in limiting progression. Although IVIG is slightly more expensive than plasmapheresis, at least in the United States, these differences in intensive care unit and hospital stay translate into enormous savings in the overall health care bill. IVIG was also better tolerated than plasmapheresis. Complications of plasmapheresis were almost twice as common as those of IVIG and tended to be more serious. Sixteen percent of patients treated with plasmapheresis had to have one or more courses stopped because of complications such as cardiovascular instability whereas none of the IVIG patients had significant adverse effects. IVIG is easier to administer and may even be effectively given subcutaneously, a factor that is extremely important in children and others, such as the elderly in whom there is poor venous access. In addition, it needs no special equipment, and requires a shorter treatment period.

Our own experience with IVIG for the treatment of GBS has also been gratifying. I particularly want to emphasize the advantages in terms of patient acceptance and safety. Treating GBS with plasmapheresis in patients who already have autonomic instability is fraught with risk and I have also found that covert autonomic instability may be unmasked by plasmapheresis. By contrast, IVIG is remarkably free of serious side effects and is extremely well tolerated. Headache is common but usually not severe and responds to reducing the rate of infusion. Similarly, tightness in the chest or overt dyspnea occasionally occurs at high infusion rates. The Dutch study found a mild rise in liver enzymes during treatment but it was never clinically significant. As with plasmapheresis, it has been suggested that relapse is more common in patients receiving IVIG but relapses respond with equal effectiveness to retreatment.[80] Nonetheless, a note of caution has been sounded by Tan and his colleagues[81] who saw two patients who developed severe renal failure during treatment with IVIG. Both had mildly elevated serum creatinine. They suggest that patients with evidence of compromised renal function should be treated with caution, using low infusion rates. We have also seen a patient with recurrent aseptic meningitis following each of two courses of IVIG[82] and cerebral thrombosis[83] has also been described. Patients with IgA deficiency should not receive IVIG as there is a significant risk of anaphylactic reaction since IVIG contains foreign IgA.[84] In the larger arena, since the introduction of the currently available forms of IVIG into the United States in 1986, there have been no reports of transmission of hepatitis, human immunodeficiency virus, or other viruses by IVIG treatment.[85]

Summary

The cornerstone of treatment for GBS remains aggressive supportive care and prevention of complications until the inevitable improvement occurs. However, in patients with rapidly progressive disease or disease of sufficient severity to prevent ambulation, plasmapheresis has proved to be safe and effective, especially if administered early. The recently published study of

IVIG suggests that it may become the treatment of choice. However, with the lack of a treatment that is entirely free of side effects and is cost effective, a search for alternatives goes on.

References

1. Brettle RP, Gross M, Legg NJ, Lockwood M, Pallis C. Treatment of acute polyneuropathy by plasma exchange. *Lancet*. 1978;2:1100.
2. Mark B, Hurwitz BJ, Olanow CW, Fay JW. Plasmapheresis in idiopathic inflammatory polyradiculoneuropathy. *Neurology*. 1980;30:361. Abstract.
3. Ropper AH, Shahani BT, Huggins CE. Improvement in 4 patients with acute Guillain-Barré syndrome after plasma exchange. *Neurology*. 1980;30:361. Abstract.
4. Rumpl E, Mayr U, Gerstenbrand F, Hackl JM, Rosmanith P, Aichner F. Treatment of Guillain-Barré syndrome by plasma exchange. *J Neurol*. 1981;225:207–217.
5. van der Heyden JE, Kennes B, Bain H, Hubert C, Neve P. Plasma exchange in acute polyneuropathy. *Acta Clin Belg*. 1979;34:246.
6. Littlewood R, Bajada S. Successful plasmapheresis in the Miller-Fisher syndrome. *Br Med J*. 1981;282:778–780.
7. Cook JD, Tindall RAS, Walker J, Khan J, Rosenberg R. Plasma exchange as a treatment of acute and chronic idiopathic autoimmune polyneuropathy: limited success. *Neurology*. 1980;30:361–362. Abstract.
8. Greenwood RJ, Newsom-Davies J, Hughes RAC, et al. Controlled trial of plasma exchange in acute inflammatory polyradiculoneuropathy. *Lancet*. 1984;1:877–879.
9. Murray NMF, Miles CM, Karni Y, Newsom-Davies J. Intensive plasma exchange in acute inflammatory polyneuropathy. *Ann Med Interne (Paris)*. 1984;135:144.
10. Osterman PO, Fagius J, Lundemo G, et al. Beneficial effects of plasma exchange in acute inflammatory polyradiculoneuropathy. *Lancet*. 1984;2:1296–1299.
11. Bezwoda WR, Fritz V, Reef HE, et al. Treatment of acute post-infective polyneuropathy by means of plasma exchange. *Acta Neurol Scand*. 1984;69:112–119.
12. Mendell JR, Kissel JT, Kennedy MS, et al. Plasma exchange and prednisone in Guillain-Barré syndrome: a controlled randomized trial. *Neurology*. 1985;35:1551–1555.
13. Cook SD, Dowling PC, Murray MR, Whitaker JN. Circulating demyelinating factors in acute idiopathic polyneuropathy. *Arch Neurol*. 1971;24:136–144.
14. Brown MJ, Rosen JL, Lisak RP. Demyelination in vivo by Guillain-Barré syndrome and other human serum. *Muscle Nerve*. 1987;10:263–271.
15. Feasby TE, Hahn AF, Gilbert JJ. Passive transfer studies in Guillain-Barré polyneuropathy. *Neurology*. 1982;32:1159–1167.
16. Harrison BM, Hansen BA, Pollard JD, McLeod LG. Demyelination induced by serum from patients with Guillain-Barré syndrome. *Ann Neurol*. 1984;15:163–170.
17. Saida T, Saida K, Lisak RP, Brown MJ, Silberberg DH, Asbury AK. In vivo demyelinating activity of sera from patients with Guillain-Barré syndrome. *Ann Neurol*. 1982;11:69–75.
18. Sumner AJ, Said G, Idy I, Metral S. Syndrome de Guillain-Barré: effets electrophysiologiques et morphologiques du serum humain introduit dans l'espace endoneurial du nerf sciatique du rat. *Rev Neurol*. 1982;138:17–24.
19. Low PA, Schmelzer JD, Dyck PJ. Results of endoneurial injection of Guillain-Barré serum in Lewis rats. *Mayo Clin Proc*. 1982;57:360–364.
20. Heininger K, Liebert UG, Toyka KV, et al. Chronic inflammatory polyneuropathy: reduction of nerve conduction velocities in monkeys by systemic passive transfer of immunoglobulins. *J Neurol Sci*. 1984;66:1–14.
21. Koski CL, Gratz E, Sutherland J, Mayer RF. Clinical correlation with anti-peripheral-nerve myelin antibodies in Guillain-Barré syndrome. *Ann Neurol*. 1986;19:573–577.
22. Metral S, Raphael JC, Hort-Legrand CI, Elkharrat D. Activite demyelinisante serique et syndrome de Guillain-Barré: effet favorable des echanges plasmatique. *Rev Neurol (Paris)*. 1989;145:312–319.
23. Rostami AM, Burns JB, Eccleston PA, Manning MC, Lisak RP, Silberberg DH. Search for antibodies to galactocerebroside in the serum and cerebrospinal fluid in human demyelinating disorders. *Ann Neurol*. 1987;22:381–383.

24. Ilyas AA, Willison HJ, Quarles RH, et al. Serum antibodies to gangliosides in Guillain-Barré syndrome. *Ann Neurol.* 1988;23:440–447.
25. The Guillain-Barré Syndrome Study Group. Plasmapheresis and acute Guillain-Barré syndrome. *Neurology.* 1985;35:1096–1104.
26. McKhann GM, Griffin JW, Cornblath DR, et al. Plasmapheresis and Guillain-Barré syndrome: analysis of prognostic factors and the effect of plasmapheresis. *Ann Neurol.* 1988; 23:347–353.
27. McKhann GM, Griffin JW, Cornblath DR, Quaskey SA, Mellitis ED. Role of therapeutic plasmapheresis in the acute Guillain-Barré syndrome. *J Neuroimmunol.* 1988;20:297–300.
28. French Cooperative Group on Plasma Exchange in Guillain-Barré Syndrome. Efficiency of plasma exchange in Guillain-Barré syndrome: role of replacement fluids. *Ann Neurol.* 1987; 22:753–761.
29. Dyck PJ, Kurtzke JF. Plasmapheresis in Guillain-Barré syndrome. *Neurology.* 1985;35:1105–1107.
30. Farkkila M, Kinnunen E, Haapanen E, Iivanainen M. Guillain-Barré syndrome: quantitative measurement of plasma exchange therapy. *Neurology.* 1987;37:837–840.
31. De Silva HJ, Gamage R, Herath HKN, Karunanayake MGS, Peiris JB. The treatment of Guillain-Barré syndrome by modified plasma exchange—a cost effective method for developing countries. *Postgrad Med J.* 1987;63:1079–1081.
32. Epstein MA, Sladky JT. The role of plasmapheresis in childhood Guillain-Barré syndrome. *Ann Neurol.* 1990;28:65–69.
33. Khatri BO, Flamini JR, Baruah JK, Dobyns WB, Konkol RJ. Plasmapheresis with acute inflammatory polyneuropathy. *Pediatr Neurol.* 1990;6:17–19.
34. Niparko N, Goldie WD, Mitchell W, Lipsey A, Snodgrass SR, Fishman L. The use of plasmapheresis in the management of Guillain-Barré syndrome in pediatric patients. *Ann Neurol.* 1989;26:448–449. Abstract.
35. Lamont PJ, Johnston HM, Berdoukas VA. Plasmapheresis in children with Guillain-Barré syndrome. *Neurology.* 1991;41:1928–1931.
36. Griesemer DA, Johnson MI. Guillain-Barré syndrome and plasmapheresis in childhood [letter]. *Ann Neurol.* 1991;29:688.
37. Jones HR, Bradshaw DY. Guillain-Barré syndrome and plasmapheresis in childhood [letter]. *Ann Neurol.* 1991;29:688–689.
38. Osterman PO, Vedeler CA, Ryberg B, Fagius J, Nyland H. Serum antibodies to peripheral nerve tissue in acute Guillain-Barré syndrome in relation to outcome of plasma exchange. *J Neurol.* 1988;235:285–289.
39. Osterman PO, Fagius J, Safwenberg J, Danielsson BG, Wikstrom B. Early relapses after plasma exchange in acute inflammatory polyradiculoneuropathy [letter]. *Lancet.* 1986;2:1161.
40. Osterman PO, Fagius J, Safwenberg J, Wikstrom B. Early relapse of acute inflammatory polyradiculoneuropathy after successful treatment with plasma exchange. *Acta Neurol Scand.* 1988;77:273–277.
41. Ropper AH, Albers JW, Addison R. Limited relapse in Guillain-Barré syndrome after plasma exchange. *Arch Neurol.* 1988;45:314–315.
42. Rudnicki S, Vriesendorp F, Koski CL, Mayer RF. Electrophysiological studies in the Guillain-Barré syndrome: effects of plasma and antibody rebound. *Muscle Nerve.* 1992;15:57–62.
43. Shy GM, McEachern D. Further studies of the effects of cortisone and ACTH on neurological disorders. *Brain.* 1951;7:354–362.
44. Plum F. Multiple symmetrical polyneuropathy treated with cortisone. *Neurology.* 1953;3:661–667.
45. Heller GL, DeJong RN. Treatment of the Guillain-Barré syndrome. Use of corticotrophin and glucocorticoids. *Arch Neurol.* 1963;8:179–193.
46. Sandu L. Corticosteroids in Landry-Guillain-Barré-Strohl syndrome. *Lancet.* 1974;2:662.
47. Frick E, Angstwurm H. Corticosteroid treatment of idiopathic polyneuritis. *Munch Med Wochenschr.* 1968;110:1265–1271.
48. Samantray SK, Johnson, SC, Mathai KV, Pulimood BM. Landry-Guillain-Barré-Strohl syndrome. A study of 302 cases. *Med J Aust.* 1977;2:84–91.
49. Wiederholt WC, Mulder DW, Lambert EH. The Landry-Guillain-Barré-Strohl syndrome or polyradiculoneuropathy: historical review, report on 97 patients, and present concepts. *Mayo Clin Proc.* 1964;39:427–451.
50. Swick HM, McQuillen MP. The use of steroids in the treatment of idiopathic polyneuritis. *Neurology.* 1976;26:205–212.

51. Hughes RAC, Newsom-Davies J, Perkin GD, Pierce JM. Controlled trial of prednisolone in acute polyneuropathy. *Lancet*. 1978;2:750–753.
52. Brumbach RA. Failure of oral versus parenteral corticosteroids in a case of acute inflammatory polyradiculoneuropathy (Guillain-Barré syndrome). *Aust NZ J Med*. 1980;10:224–226.
53. Dowling PC, Bosch VV, Cook SD. Possible beneficial effect of high-dose intravenous steroid therapy in acute demyelinating disease and transverse myelitis. *Neurology*. 1980;30:33–36.
54. Haab A, Trabert W, Grebnich N, Schimrigk K. High-dose steroid therapy in Guillain-Barré syndrome. *J Neuroimmunol*. 1988;20:305–308.
55. Hughes RAC. Ineffectiveness of high-dose intravenous methylprednisolone in Guillain-Barré syndrome. *Lancet*. 1991;338:1142.
56. Drachman DA, Paterson PY, Berling BS, Roguska J. Immunosuppression and the Guillain-Barré syndrome. *Arch Neurol*. 1970;23:385–393.
57. Grant H, Leopold HN. Guillain-Barré syndrome occurring during cortisone therapy. *JAMA*. 1954;155:252–253.
58. Steiner I, Wirguin I, Abramsky O. Appearance of Guillain-Barré syndrome in patients during corticosteroid treatment. *J Neurol*. 1986;233:221–223.
59. Preston DC, Logigian EL. Guillain-Barré syndrome during high-dose methylprednisolone therapy [letter]. *Muscle Nerve*. 1991;14:378–379.
60. King RHM, Craggs RI, Gross MLP, Tompkins C, Thomas PK. Suppression of experimental allergic neuritis by cyclosporin-A. *Acta Neuropathol*. 1983;59:262–268.
61. Levine S, Sowinski R. Suppression of the hyperacute form of experimental allergic encephalomyelitis by drugs. *Arch Int Pharmacodyn*. 1977;230:309–318.
62. Palmer KNV. Polyradiculoneuropathy (Guillain-Barré syndrome) treated with 6-mercaptopurine. *Lancet*. 1965;1:733–734.
63. Palmer KNV. Polyradiculoneuropathy treated with cytotoxic drugs [letter]. *Lancet*. 1966; 1:265.
64. Colin-Jones DG, Heathfield KWG. 6-mercaptopurine in polyradiculoneuropathy [letter]. *Lancet*. 1965;2:739.
65. Yuill GM, Swinburn WR, Liversedge LA. Treatment of polyneuropathy with azathioprine. *Lancet*. 1970;2:854–856.
66. Rosen AD, Vastola EF. Clinical effects of cyclophosphamide in Guillain-Barré polyneuritis. *J Neurol Sci*. 1976;30:179–187.
67. Roifman CM, Schaffer FM, Wachsmuth SE, Murphy G, Gelfand EW. Reversal of chronic polymyositis following intravenous immune serum globulin therapy. *JAMA*. 1987;258: 513–515.
68. Fehr J, Hofmann V, Kappelee V. Transient reversal of thrombocytopenia in idiopathic thrombocytopenic purpura by high-dose intravenous gamma globulin. *N Engl J Med*. 1982; 356:1254–1258.
69. Gelfand EW. The use of intravenous immune globulin in collagen vascular disorders: a potentially new modality of therapy. *J Allergy Clin Immunol*. 1989;84:613–616.
70. Faed JM, Day B, Pollock M, Taylor PK, Nukada H, Hammond-Tooke GD. High-dose intravenous human immunoglobulin in chronic inflammatory demyelinating polyneuropathy. *Neurology*. 1989;39:422–425.
71. van Doorn PA, Brand A, Strengers PFW, Meulstee J, Vermeulen M. High-dose intravenous immunoglobulin treatment in chronic inflammatory demyelinating polyneuropathy: a double-blind, placebo-controlled, crossover study. *Neurology*. 1990;40:209–212.
72. Kleyweg RP, van der Meche FGA, Meulstee J. Treatment of Guillain-Barré syndrome with high-dose gammaglobulin. *Neurology*. 1988;38:1639–1641.
73. Mauro G. Un case de syndrome de Guillain-Barré tratie par forte doses d'immunoglobulines par voie intraveineuse. *Rev Neurol (Paris)*. 1989;145:731–732.
74. Shahar E, Murphy EG, Roifman CM. Beneficial effect of high-dose intravenous gamma globulin in severe Guillain-Barré syndrome. *Ann Neurol*. 1989;26:448. Abstract.
75. Shahar E, Murphy EG, Roifman CM. Benefit of intravenously administered immune serum globulin in patients with Guillain-Barré syndrome. *J Pediatr*. 1990;116:141–144.
76. Lavenstein B, Sirdofsky M, Watkin T. High-dose IV gamma globulin therapy in childhood Guillain-Barré syndrome. *Neurology*. 1990;40:408–400. Abstract.
77. Jackson AH, Donnelly JH. The efficacy of high-dose intravenous gammaglobulin in the treatment of Guillain-Barré syndrome in childhood. *Ann Neurol*. 1990;28:431. Abstract.
78. van der Meche FGA, Kleyweg RP, Meulstee J, Oomes PG. High-dose intravenous gammaglobulin in Guillain-Barré syndrome [letter]. *Ann Neurol*. 1988;24:588.

79. van der Meche FGA, Schmitz PIM and the Dutch Guillain-Barré Study Group. A randomized trial comparing intravenous immune globulin and plasma exchange in Guillain-Barré syndrome. *N Engl J Med.* 1992;326:1123–1129.

80. Kleyweg RP, van der Meche FGA. Treatment related fluctuations in Guillain-Barré syndrome after high-dose immunoglobulins or plasma-exchange. *J Neurol Neurosurg Psychiatry.* 1991; 54:957–960.

81. Tan E, Hajinazarian MO, Bay W, Mendell JR. Acute renal failure: serious complication of immunoglobulin G (IVIG) treatment. *Neurology.* 1992;42(suppl 3):335. Abstract.

82. Vera-Ramirez M, Charlet M, Parry GJ. Recurrent aseptic meningitis complicating intravenous immunoglobulin therapy for chronic inflammatory polyradiculoneuropathy. *Neurology.* 1992;42:1636–1637.

83. Silbert PL, Knezevic WV, Bridge BT. Cerebral infarction complicating intravenous immunoglobulin therapy for polyneuritis cranialis. *Neurology.* 1992;42:257–258.

84. McCluskey DR, Boyd NAM. Anaphylaxis with intravenous gammaglobulin [letter]. *Lancet.* 1990;2:874.

85. Schwartz RS. Overview of the biochemistry and safety of a new native intravenous gamma globulin, IGIV, pH 4.25. *Am J Med.* 1987;83(suppl 4A):46–56.

7

Epidemiology of Guillain-Barré Syndrome

Epidemiological studies can provide important insights to disease, particularly those for which the exact etiology is obscure. By evaluating the entire population of a well defined geographic area, epidemiologists can determine the frequency of a particular disease at a given time (disease prevalence). By determining the number of new cases that occur during a specified time interval, the disease incidence can be ascertained. The mortality can be calculated from the number of deaths occurring from the disease during a particular time interval. In addition, the association of a disease with antecedent or concurrent events may provide important clues to its etiology. The utility of these parameters depends on the accuracy of the diagnosis and the methods of case ascertainment. With a heterogeneous disorder like neuropathy this is a major confounding problem. However, the acute evolution of GBS and the relative paucity of diseases that mimic it enhance diagnostic accuracy. Nonetheless, many mild cases are undoubtedly missed and even severe cases may be misdiagnosed. These caveats must be borne in mind when evaluating epidemiological data.

Incidence of Guillain-Barré Syndrome

Although a rare disease, Guillain-Barré syndrome (GBS) occurs worldwide and affects all ages and races. The reported incidence ranges from 0.6 to 1.9 cases per 100,000 persons per year.[1–12] This wide variation almost certainly

113

relates to differences in methods of case collection rather than to true differences in incidence in different areas. The higher incidences are usually reported from intensive studies of small, well defined populations, where mild cases are more likely to be detected. A much higher incidence was reported from Larimer County, Colorado, for the 3-year period beginning in 1981.[13] During that time 19 new cases were reported, giving an incidence of 4.0 per 100,000 per year compared with an incidence of 1.2 per 100,000 per year from 1975 to 1980. Surrounding counties had no such increase in incidence. No particular predisposing features were identified and the disease characteristics were no different. The explanation for this increased incidence remains obscure and it may simply represent biological variation.

About 70% of GBS cases follow an identifiable febrile illness and yet, in most studies, there has not been a recognizable seasonal preponderance despite the increased occurrence of febrile illnesses in certain seasons. Baoxun et al.[14] in Beijing noted an increased incidence in the late summer and early fall (July–October), which they attributed to the increased frequency of enteric infections at that time of year. However, the accuracy of the diagnosis of many of those cases has been called into question, given the lack of sophisticated technology such as high quality electrodiagnostic testing. Many of these cases, particularly those occurring in children and young adults, may have been examples of the recently described acute paralytic illness, thought to be a reversible motor neuron disease.[15,16] These patients bear a striking clinical resemblance to patients with GBS with a preceding prodromal illness, an acutely evolving paralysis and areflexia, and occasional bulbar and respiratory failure. About half have elevated cerebrospinal fluid (CSF) protein with albuminocytologic dissociation. That the true incidence of GBS in this population is probably much lower is supported by the finding that, of 23 patients with acute paralysis in whom electrodiagnostic studies were performed, only 2 had findings indicative of GBS.[16] Dowling et al.[17,18] also noted an increased frequency of cases arising in the late summer and fall in the New York–Northern New Jersey region and related these to an increased incidence of cytomegalovirus (CMV) infection occurring at that time. Lassen and Fog,[19] Petlund,[20] Ravn,[21] and Larsen et al.[22] also noted a small excess of cases in the fall.

Although GBS is usually a sporadic disease occurring throughout the year, there have been several identifiable outbreaks where numbers of cases recognized exceeded the expected incidence by 20 to 400 times. In 1968 there was an outbreak in Colombia for which no identifiable precipitant was identified.[23] Two outbreaks occurred in 1976. One occurred in Jordan and followed an epidemic of more than 5000 cases of acute diarrhea.[24] No single triggering infection was identified but several patients had typhoid or hepatitis virus infection. The second outbreak in 1976, which will be discussed in more detail below, occurred after the immunization of approximately 45 million people against swine influenza in the United States. There have been two outbreaks of GBS in South America after rabies vaccination.[25,26] In one, the incidence of this complication fell sharply when the dose of vaccine was reduced.[25] Finally, there were two outbreaks in 1985. One occurred in Finland after a nationwide vaccination program against poliomyelitis.[27,28] The other occurred in Japan with no recognized cause.[29] The latter was curious for its high incidence of ophthalmoplegia.

Although no age group is immune, the disease is rare in children, particularly during the first 2 years of life, and tends to increase in frequency throughout life, although there is a small peak in frequency in young adult life.[6] In one recent study, the annual incidence in children under 15 years of age was 0.38 per 100,000[30] whereas in adults older than 60 years it is 3.2 per 100,000. The lack of a more distinct preponderance of cases in young adults is curious for a presumptive autoimmune disease since most are more common in young adult life and become less common with increasing age. In most surveys, the incidence is only slightly higher for men and in whites, although in one Minnesota study[31] men outnumbered women by almost 2:1.

Because there is a predisposition for many immunological conditions to develop in individuals with certain histocompatibility antigens, many people have sought a common antigen or group of antigens in patients with GBS. In the relapsing and progressive chronic inflammatory demyelinating neuropathies (CIDP) there is an increased incidence of HLA AW30, AW31, A1, B8, and DRw3,[32–35] but these same antigens have not been associated with GBS. However, a genetic influence on the susceptibility to demyelinating diseases of both the central and peripheral nervous systems has been demonstrated. GBS, CIDP, and multiple sclerosis have all been shown to be associated with the presence of the M3 allele of the alpha-1-antitrypsin system, located on chromosome 14.[36] In addition, Gm haplotypes, which are closely linked to alpha-1-antitrypsin on chromosome 14 and code for constant regions of immunoglobulin, are found with increased frequency in patients with GBS and, to a lesser extent, in patients with CIDP.[37]

Antecedent Events and Associated Illnesses

GBS After Infections

GBS often is associated with an antecedent illness, usually an acute non-specific infection (Table 7–1). The incidence of preceding infection as reported in different series ranges from 52%[38] to 80%[39] (Table 7–2). Neurological symptoms may begin as much as 4 weeks later, although in most patients the onset is much sooner with the mean interval, compiled from several different series, being 12 days.[7,39–42] The possibility of much longer incubation periods was put forward by Poser and Behan.[43] They suggested that the delay may be as much as weeks or even months although, in isolated cases with such long incubation periods, it is not possible to establish with certainty a relationship between the antecedent event and the neuropathy. However,

Table 7–1. Antecedent Events and Associated Illnesses

Infection
Vaccination
Surgery
Systemic illnesses
  Malignancy
  Systemic lupus erythematosus
  Renal transplantation
  Thyroiditis
  Addison's disease

during epidemics of GBS occurring in association with vaccination programs, such as the swine influenza program in the United States in 1976 and the poliomyelitis vaccination program in Finland in 1985, clustering of cases strongly suggests a common antecedent event. In both of these epidemics a latent interval of at least 12 weeks occurred in some cases. One consistent observation is that there is an inverse relationship between severity of the neurological illness and the duration of the latent period. That is, with the shorter incubation periods the neurological illness is more severe. In their report of 50 severe cases resulting in death, Haymaker and Kernohan[39] noted that in some, the neurological illness began during the acute or subacute phase of the prodrome or within the first week thereafter and, conversely, in the cases with a very long latent period such as those reported by Poser and Behan,[43] the neurological disease ran a benign course.

In most cases, the antecedent infection has resolved by the time the neurological symptoms appear. However, several viral infections that have been associated with the subsequent development of GBS are notoriously

Table 7–2. Infections Associated with GBS

	DEFINITE	PROBABLE	POSSIBLE
Viral	CMV EBV	HIV Varicella-zoster Vaccinia/smallpox	Influenza Measles Mumps Rubella Hepatitis Coxsackie Echo

Bacterial	*Campylobacter
	    jejuni*
	*Mycoplasma
	    pneumonia*
		Typhoid (some
		    epidemics)
			Borrelia burgdorferi (Lyme disease)
			Paratyphoid
			Brucellosis
			Chlamydia
			Legionella
			Listeria

chronic, and evidence of persistent infection may still be apparent at the time of onset of the neurological illness. For example, the occasional persistent CSF pleocytosis may represent a resolving subclinical or oligosymptomatic meningoencephalitis associated with the prodromal illness. This applies most notably to infection with CMV, Epstein-Barr virus (EBV), human immunodeficiency virus (HIV), and *Borrelia burgdorferi* (Lyme disease), although occasional persistence of CSF pleocytosis is seen with unidentified and nonspecific prodromes. Most commonly, patients describe the preceding illness as a mild upper respiratory infection or gastroenteritis, the cause of which is seldom identified.[44]

GBS AFTER VIRAL INFECTIONS

Occasionally GBS may follow a defined viral infectious illness. The most commonly identified associated infection is with CMV, which can cause a number of clinical syndromes including upper respiratory infections, gastroenteritis, and a syndrome with clinical features similar to infectious mononucleosis. In one study, there was serological evidence of recent CMV infection in 15% of cases.[17,18] Most reported an upper respiratory illness and some had fever, malaise, headache, and gastroenteritis. However, 20% of those with serological evidence of a recent infection did not recall a recent symptomatic illness. GBS has also been associated with renal transplantation.[45] Although it appears paradoxical that GBS, a presumptive autoimmune neuropathy, should occur in these profoundly immunosuppressed patients, it is noteworthy that they are frequently infected with CMV, perhaps explaining the frequency with which GBS occurs.[45,46] CMV has occasionally been identified within the peripheral nerves in immunocompromised patients. Typical CMV inclusions were found in spinal roots and peripheral nerves of a patient with GBS who was immunosuppressed after renal transplantation.[47] CMV inclusions were also found in Schwann cells in lumbar dorsal roots and in the lumbosacral plexus in two patients with AIDS who developed GBS.[48] These cases raise the possibility that some cases of GBS may result from virus-induced demyelination or from an immune-mediated attack on CMV-infected Schwann cells.

GBS is also commonly associated with infectious mononucleosis due to EBV infection.[49-54] With EBV infection there is commonly an associated encephalopathy that may cause diagnostic confusion.[55,56] The onset of weakness may be attributed to central nervous system (CNS) involvement and, conversely, encephalopathy may be attributed to GBS and used as evidence of central involvement. Both EBV and CMV are herpes viruses and Marek's disease, another spontaneous inflammatory demyelinating neuropathy that occurs in fowl,[57,58] is also caused by a herpes virus. Another herpes virus with which an association with GBS has been suggested is the varicella-zoster virus.[59-61] Although GBS is uncommon in children, there have been several reports of GBS after chicken pox in children, the number of cases exceeding that which would be expected in children. There have also been a number of cases of GBS after herpes zoster,[62-64] but this relationship is somewhat more tenuous. However, the bulk of the evidence suggests that there is an increased frequency of GBS occurring after infection with the varicella-zoster virus. An association with herpes simplex infection[65] has also been suggested but is even more difficult to prove than varicella-zoster since the former is so ubiquitous. This intriguing association between herpes virus infections and GBS suggests that they may have a particular predilection for triggering demyelination of peripheral nerves.[66] An association of GBS with smallpox and with vaccination against smallpox with vaccinia virus[67-69] is also highly likely, although the virtual eradication of smallpox and the disappearance of vaccination programs make it impossible to evaluate the relationship using modern methods. Vaccinia-associated GBS appears to be more common after revaccination.

GBS has been described in association with all of the various stages of HIV infection in adults[70-72] and children.[73] It may occur after the initial acute HIV infection,[74,75] as the presenting feature of otherwise asymptomatic infection,[76,77] associated with AIDS-related complex (ARC) and the lymphadenopathy syndrome (LAS),[71-73] and occasionally with established AIDS.[77-80] However, it occurs more frequently with asymptomatic infection or ARC/LAS than in patients with fully developed AIDS. That is, GBS is much more likely to occur at a time when the patient is still capable of mounting an immunological response and becomes much less likely as the immune system becomes progressively compromised. Clinically and electrophysiologically, HIV-associated GBS is indistinguishable from any other form. However, a CSF lymphocytic pleocytosis is almost invariable at the time of presentation of the neuropathy and is usually persistent. The pattern of peripheral nerve demyelination occurring in some severely immunosuppressed AIDS patients with demyelinating neuropathy is different from that in patients with minimal immune suppression. In many patients the neuropathy appears to run a much more indolent course and is not associated with inflammation, suggesting that it may have a different pathogenesis and may be virus-induced.[80] HIV-infected patients are almost always coinfected with CMV, raising the possibility that the stimulus to this more indolent form of demyelination may be the result of the CMV infection since it is so commonly associated with GBS. However, occasionally in severely immune compromised HIV-infected patients the neuropathy runs an acute course characteristic of typical GBS.

A relationship between GBS and numerous other spontaneous viral infections, including measles, rubella, mumps, hepatitis A and B, echovirus, cocksackie virus, influenza virus A and B, respiratory syncitial virus, and others has been suggested but the associations have not been established with certainty.[44] An acute ascending paralysis with inflammatory, macrophage-mediated demyelination of peripheral nerves has even been described in patients with Creutzfeldt-Jakob disease.[81,82] Josiphov has suggested that the demyelination may be due to infection of Schwann cells with the infectious agent.[82] Despite the documented association of GBS with one vaccination program for influenza, there is not an established increased risk of developing GBS after naturally acquired influenza. Most patients in whom GBS develops after a clearly identifiable antecedent infection are young and, conversely, the chances of identifying the cause of the preceding infection in the elderly is remote.

GBS AFTER BACTERIAL INFECTIONS

GBS is rarely associated with bacterial infections. A notable exception is the relationship to infection with mycoplasma pneumoniae,[83–85] an organism notorious for triggering other immunological disorders, some of them neurological (acute disseminated encephalomyelitis, acute cerebellar ataxia). As with specifically identified viral infections, these patients are mainly young. An association with typhoid fever[86] has also been suggested and one outbreak of GBS occurred in the Middle East after an epidemic gastroenteritis, many cases of which were identified as typhoid.[24]

Recently, a high proportion of GBS patients with and without diarrhea have been shown to have serological evidence of recent infection with *Campylobacter jejuni*, a gram-negative bacterium that is one of the most frequent causes of gastroenteritis.[87–91] It has been suggested that this bacterium has a particular propensity for precipitating GBS. The risk for developing GBS with *Campylobacter* infection seems to be confined to infection with the type 19 serotype.[92] In some studies,[92–94] no clinical, electrophysiological, or serological differences were found between GBS patients with *Campylobacter* antibodies and those without. Others have suggested that patients with *Campylobacter* antibodies are more likely to have antibodies to GM-1 ganglioside[95] and have more severe axonal degeneration and therefore a worse prognosis.[96,97] A rationale for the propensity of *Campylobacter* to cause GBS was put forward by Fujimoto and Amako.[98] They found that antiserum raised in mice against *C. jejuni* isolated from a GBS patient reacted strongly with the myelin-specific protein P0 and weakly with P2, suggesting that *C. jejuni* contains a protein with antigenic properties similar to myelin-specific proteins. Oomes et al.[95] found that GM1 ganglioside antibodies in the serum of patients with GBS recognized epitopes on the *Campylobacter* bacterium and suggested that molecular mimickry between *Campylobacter* and host tissue might lead to antibody-mediated demyelination. The exact relationship between *Campylobacter* infection and the subsequent development of GBS remains to be fully elucidated.

There have been several reports of GBS occurring in association with Lyme disease, which is caused by the spirochete *Borrelia burgdorferi*.[99–102] Between 30% and 40% of patients with Lyme disease have clinical and electrophysiological evidence of neuropathy, but in most it is chronic and primarily axonal in type. In those patients with demyelinating neuropathy, most are also chronic, but several cases of acutely evolving neuropathy with clinical and electrophysiological features characteristic of GBS have also been described. Most of these patients are somewhat atypical, but only insofar as they have a persistent CSF pleocytosis associated with the increased CSF protein. However, two patients with GBS and the typical albuminocytologic dissociation were described by Bouma and Carpay.[103] Neither patient had other neurological or systemic manifestations of Lyme disease and both responded to antibiotic treatment. This report underscores the importance of testing for Lyme disease in patients with GBS, at least in endemic areas. Patients with Lyme disease have increased levels of circulating IgM that cross-react with axons but binding to myelin has not been reported. GBS in patients infected with *B. burgdorferi* evolves in the usual acute fashion and should be treated in the same way as any other GBS case. However, patients should also receive treatment for the underlying infection with penicillin or other appropriate antibiotics. GBS has also been reported after paratyphoid fever,[104] brucellosis,[105] chlamydial infection,[106] Legionnaires' disease,[107] listeriosis,[108] tularemia,[109] and other bacterial infections, but the numbers are too small for a causative relationship to be established with certainty.

GBS after Vaccination

GBS may also follow certain types of vaccination (Table 7–3). Shortly after the introduction of rabies vaccination by Pasteur in the late 1890s, it was soon realized that a variety of neurological complications occurred, including acute polyneuritis. This complication was related to contamination of the vaccine with neural tissue and has virtually disappeared with the introduction of vaccine prepared from duck or chick embryos. However, vaccine prepared from neural tissue is still used, particularly in underdeveloped countries; Cabrera et al.[26] described five cases of GBS after rabies vaccination in Peru. Their cases differed from typical GBS in terms of a high incidence of severe cranial nerve involvement and unusually severe disease with high mortality. In addition, their patients developed GBS during the course of immunization, indicating a short latent period between the immunological challenge and the antibody-directed response. Arnason[44] noted that rabies vaccine–associated GBS did not differ from other forms in any substantive way, although he also noted that early onset of disease was associated with a particularly severe course. The antigen in rabies vaccines that induces GBS

Table 7–3.   **Vaccinations Associated with GBS**

Definite	Rabies*
	Swine influenza†
Possible	Poliovirus
	H. influenzae
	Typhoid
	Tetanus toxoid

*Only with vaccine prepared from neural tissue.
†Only with the 1976–77 swine A/influenza vaccine.

appears to be myelin basic protein (MBP). Hemachudha et al.[110] found that 100% of the patients with postvaccinial GBS associated with the Semple rabies vaccine prepared from mature animal brains, and 20% (1/5) receiving vaccine prepared from suckling mouse brains, had antibodies to MBP but not to P2, another distinct myelin-associated protein. However, no case of idiopathic GBS had MBP or P2 antibodies, indicating that different target antigens may precipitate the immune-mediated demyelination.

The association of GBS with the swine influenza vaccination program of 1976 is also established beyond reasonable doubt.[10,111–113] In the fall of that year, approximately 50 million people in the United States were vaccinated in a program sponsored by the federal government with a vaccine containing A/New Jersey swine influenza virus. In the months that followed there was a marked increase in the frequency with which GBS occurred in patients receiving the vaccine. Between October 1, 1976 and January 31, 1977, there were 1098 patients with GBS reported to the Centers for Disease Control (CDC). Of these, 532 had received the vaccine before the onset of GBS. This represented a more than 20-fold increase in the number of cases expected to occur in nonvaccinated individuals. Before that time, only three cases of GBS associated with influenza vaccine had been reported despite the widespread incorporation of swine influenza virus in vaccines administered to military personnel in the 1950s and 1960s. Furthermore, a subsequent vaccination program in 1978–1979, using a trivalent vaccine not containing swine influenza virus, caused no increase in the expected incidence of GBS.[113] Therefore, the risk of developing GBS after influenza vaccination is unable to be predicted with accuracy since the constituents of the vaccine are obviously important. At the moment it seems prudent to avoid the use of vaccines containing swine influenza virus.

GBS may also occur after vaccination with live attenuated poliovirus.[27,28] During 1985, after an outbreak of poliomyelitis in Finland, 94% of the population of that country was vaccinated with live, attenuated, poliovirus vaccine over a 5-week period. In the district of Uusimaa in southern Finland, there was a marked increase in the number of GBS cases seen over the next 4 months. It is possible that some previous cases of paralytic illnesses reported after poliovirus vaccination and attributed to vaccine-related poliomyelitis may have been unrecognized GBS.

The association between GBS and other types of vaccination is less well established. There is a single report of GBS occurring in three children, one week after vaccination against Hemophilus influenzae.[114] The temporal relationship and the occurrence in more than one child suggests that the relationship may be causative. There have also been reports of GBS after vaccination against typhoid, in which the onset of the neuropathy coincided with a local reaction at the site of injection, suggesting that both were related to a generalized host response. Rare cases of GBS after tetanus inoculation have also been described and, in one case, acute demyelinating neuropathy developed on three separate occasions after tetanus toxoid injection.[115] Treatment of blepharospasm with another *Clostridium* toxin, namely botulinum toxin, has also been followed by GBS.[116] Cases of GBS after vaccination against measles, rubella, and with the DPT vaccine of childhood have also been described, but there are insufficient data to establish a definite association.

GBS after Surgery

About 5% of GBS cases may follow surgery.[44,117,118] There is no particular association with surgery at specific sites or for specific illnesses. GBS has been described after surgery to the cranium, thorax, abdomen, and limbs. In some cases the surgery has been complicated by infection but others have been uncomplicated. Cases have been described using either spinal or general anesthesia, and they may also be associated with hyperalimentation. Steiner et al.[119] reported four cases of GBS after spinal epidural anesthesia and suggested that nerve root injury might be the factor that triggered the neuropathy. However, it is impossible to separate the possible triggering effect of surgery from the preceding anesthesia. It has been suggested that GBS after surgery tends to be particularly severe.[44]

GBS Associated with Pregnancy

GBS does occur during pregnancy but the association seems to be no more than fortuitous.[120] It may occur during any trimester or during the puerperium. The course of the disease does not appear to be affected by the pregnancy, by abortion or by parturition. There have been no reports of fetal involvement.

GBS with Malignancy and Other Systemic Diseases

GBS may also occur in association with Hodgkin's disease and other reticuloses and occasionally with other malignancies.[121-124] There have been several reports of a Guillain-Barré–like illness associated with sarcoidosis.[125-127] In most cases the evolution is slower, over several weeks, and the CSF is usually cellular and may have hypoglycorrhachia. GBS has also been described in association with circulating immune complexes and in one case there was a coincident immune complex nephritis.[128,129] Acute demyelinating neuropathy may also be seen in patients with systemic lupus erythematosis.[130] It tends to run a somewhat slower course than classical GBS, but it is otherwise indistinguishable. Occasional cases of GBS have also been reported in association with Hashimoto's thyroiditis, hyperthyroidism and Addison's disease,[44] all conditions associated with demonstrated abnormalities of cell-mediated immunity, as well as with alpha-1-antitrypsin deficiency.[131]

There have been recent anecdotal reports from Germany of GBS after treatment of other neurological disorders with ganglioside mixtures. However, several hundred thousand patients have been treated in other countries without any increase in the incidence of associated GBS, suggesting that the association is purely coincidental.

GBS Associated with Drugs

There have been several reports of GBS occurring in association with the therapeutic use of drugs as well as with illicit drug use. The infrequency of the association casts doubt on any pathogenetic role. On some occasions, the GBS may be related to the underlying disease for which the drug is being used rather than to the drug itself. There are many reports of neuropathy complicating gold therapy for rheumatoid arthritis but in most it is not an acute inflammatory demyelinating neuropathy.[132] However, typical GBS[133] as well as Miller-Fisher syndrome[134] have been described with gold therapy. Simultaneous onset of both GBS and pemphigus foliaceus, an immunological disorder of skin, has been described after treatment with D-penicillamine for rheumatoid arthritis.[135] Penicillamine can also precipitate myasthenia gravis, another autoimmune neurological disease. GBS has also been rarely described in association with myasthenia gravis.[136,137] It has been suggested that certain patients may inherit a predisposition to the development of these two autoimmune diseases since the chance association of two such rare conditions has been calculated at one per two billion people per year.[137] GBS has also been described after treatment with streptokinase,[138–141] captopril,[142,143] danazol,[144] and zimeldine,[145] and after overdose with amitriptyline.[146] Several cases of acute neuropathy, some resembling GBS, have also been described after intravenous heroin use.[147–150]

Mechanism of Triggering Events

The mechanisms whereby infection, vaccinations, trauma, and other factors may trigger acute demyelination in GBS are not known with certainty. In some instances, such as rabies vaccination, it seems that inoculation of neural antigens from vaccinations prepared in neural tissues provides the stimulus for subsequent antibody-mediated demyelination of the peripheral nerves. In support of this hypothesis is the observation that preparation of rabies vaccines in chick embryos appears to have eliminated rabies vaccine–induced GBS. A possible mechanism for GBS associated with viral infections is virus-induced demyelination. Virtually all of the viruses associated with GBS are neurotropic and it is conceivable that direct invasion of Schwann cells could result in myelin damage. However, it is unlikely that such a wide variety of different viruses could produce such a stereotyped response. Furthermore, demyelination would be expected to occur during the acute phase of the infection rather than with a latent period of days to weeks. It is more likely that a variety of viruses or, for that matter, any infection or vaccination, can trigger an immune response that becomes directed against components of peripheral nerve myelin. Invading organisms may share antigenic similarity with myelin antigens and the antibody response induced by the invader may spill over into an attack on normal myelin. In some instances, such as with CMV and possibly other viruses, viral infection of Schwann cells may result in an antibody attack on the cell containing the virus, leading to myelin damage. Malignant and autoimmune diseases may similarly produce antibodies that cross-react with myelin. Trauma may trigger demyelination by releasing previously sequestered myelin antigens into the circulation and exciting an immunological response directed against myelin.

Summary

GBS is an acute, demyelinating neuropathy occurring with roughly equal frequency in males and females of all ages and races and in all areas of the world. About 70% of cases follow a recognized infection, usually viral, or are associated with some other identifiable antecedent event. Although it is usually sporadic, without a particular seasonal preponderance, several epidemics have occurred, after vaccination programs or spontaneously. The exact mechanisms that result in acute, monophasic demyelination, confined to peripheral nerves, are uncertain but the temporal association with infections and vaccinations supports the concept that GBS is an immunological disorder.

References

1. Bak P. Guillain-Barré syndrome in a Danish county. *Neurology*. 1985;35:207–211.
2. Brewis M, Poskanzer DC, Rolland H. Neurological disease in an English city. *Acta Neurol Scand*. 1966;42(suppl 24):1–89.
3. Chen K, Brody JA, Kurland LT. Patterns of neurologic diseases on Guam. I. Epidemiologic aspects. *Arch Neurol*. 1968;19:573–578.
4. Gudmundsson KR. Prevalence and occurrence of some rare neurological diseases in Iceland. *Acta Neurol Scand*. 1969;45:114–118.
5. Hogg JE, Kobrin DE, Schoenberg BS. The Guillain-Barré syndrome: epidemiologic and clinical features. *J Chronic Dis*. 1979;32:227–231.
6. Kennedy RH, Danielson MA, Mulder DW, Kurland LT. Guillain-Barré syndrome. A 42 year epidemiologic and clinical study. *Mayo Clin Proc*. 1978;53:93–99.
7. Masucci EF, Kurtzke JG. Diagnostic criteria for the Guillain-Barré syndrome. An analysis of 50 cases. *J Neurol Sci*. 1971;13:483–501.
8. Nyland H. Epidemiology of Guillain-Barré syndrome in mid-Western Norway. *Acta Neurol Scand*. 1978;57(suppl 67):223.
9. Radhakrishnan K, el-Mangoush MA, Gerryo SE. Descriptive epidemiology of selected neuromuscular disorders in Benghazi, Libya. *Acta Neurol Scand*. 1987;75:95–100.
10. Schonberger LB, Hurwitz ES, Katona P, Holman RC, Bregman DJ. Guillain-Barré syndrome: its epidemiology and associations with influenza vaccination. *Ann Neurol*. 1981;9(suppl):31–38.
11. Soffer D, Feldman S, Alter M. Epidemiology of Guillain-Barré syndrome. *Neurology*. 1978;28:686–690.

12. Storey E, Cook M. Peppard R, Newton-John H, Byrne E. Guillain-Barré syndrome and related conditions in Victorian teaching hospitals 1980–84. *Aust NZ J Med.* 1989;19:687–693.
13. Kaplan JE, Poduska PJ, McIntosh GC, Hopkins RS, Ferguson SW, Schonberger LB. Guillain-Barré syndrome in Larimer County, Colorado: a high-incidence area. *Neurology.* 1985;35:581–584.
14. Baoxun Z, Yinchang Y, Huifen H, Xiuqin L. Acute polyradiculitis (Guillain-Barré syndrome): an epidemiological study of 156 cases observed in Beijing. *Ann Neurol.* 1981;9 (suppl):146–148.
15. McKhann GM, Cornblath DR, Ho T, et al. Acute paralytic disease of children and young adults in Northern China. *Ann Neurol.* 1991;30:260. Abstract.
16. Cornblath DR, McKhann GM, Ho T, et al. Electrophysiology of acute paralytic disease of children and young adults in Northern China. *Ann Neurol.* 1991;30:260. Abstract.
17. Dowling PC, Menonna JP, Cook SD. Guillain-Barré syndrome in Greater New York-New Jersey. *JAMA.* 1977;238:317–318.
18. Dowling PC, Cook SD. Role of infection in Guillain-Barré syndrome: laboratory confirmation of herpesvirus in 41 cases. *Ann Neurol.* 1981;9(suppl):44–55.
19. Lassen HCA, Fog M. Acute polyradiculitis. *Acta Med Scand.* 1943;115:117–138.
20. Petlund CF. Polyradiculitis Guillain-Barré et 10-ars-materiale. (Review of 10 years LGBS cases). *T Norske Laegeforen.* 1962;82:1139–1141.
21. Ravn H. The Landry-Guillain-Barré syndrome. A survey and clinical report of 127 cases. *Acta Neurol Scand.* 1967;43:(suppl 30):1–64.
22. Larsen JP, Kvale G, Nyland H. Epidemiology of Guillain-Barré syndrome in the county of Hordaland, Western Norway. *Acta Neurol Scand.* 1985;71:43–47.
23. Lopez F, Lopez JH, Holguin J, Flewett TH. An acute outbreak of acute polyradiculoneuropathy in Colombia in 1968. *Am J Epidemiol.* 1973;98:226–230.
24. Sliman NA. Outbreak of Guillain-Barré syndrome associated with water pollution. *Br Med J.* 1978;1:751–752.
25. Toro G, Vergara I, Roman G. Neuroparalytic accidents of antirabies vaccination with suckling mouse brain vaccine. Clinical and pathologic study of 21 cases. *Arch Neurol.* 1977;34:694–700.
26. Carbrera J, Griffin DE, Johnson RT. Unusual features of the Guillain-Barré syndrome after rabies vaccine prepared in suckling mouse brain. *J Neurol Sci.* 1987;81:239–245.
27. Kinnunen E, Farkkila M, Hovi T, Juntunen J, Weckstrom P. Incidence of Guillain-Barré syndrome during a nationwide oral poliovirus vaccine campaign. *Neurology.* 1989;39:1034–1036.
28. Uhari M, Rantala H, Niemel M. Cluster of childhood Guillain-Barré cases after an oral poliovaccine campaign. *Lancet.* 1989;2:440–441.
29. Kashihara K, Yabuki S, Mimori Y, Yamazaki M, Yamashita M. An outbreak of Guillain-Barré syndrome with ophthalmoplegia in Kochi. *Rinsho Shinkeigaku.* 1987;27:305–309.
30. Rantala H, Uhari M, Niemala M. Occurrence, clinical manifestations, and prognosis of Guillain-Barré syndrome. *Arch Dis Child.* 1991;66:706–709.
31. Beghi E, Kurland LT, Mulder DW, Wiederholt WC. Guillain-Barré syndrome: clinicoepidemiologic features and effect of influenza vaccine. *Arch Neurol.* 1985;42:1053–1057.
32. Adams D, Festenstein H, Gibson JD, et al. HLA antigens in chronic relapsing idiopathic inflammatory polyneuropathy. *J Neurol Neurosurg Psychiatry.* 1979;42:184–186.
33. Adams D, Gibson JD, Thomas PK, et al. HLA antigens in Guillain-Barré syndrome. *Lancet.* 1977;2:504–505.
34. Latovitski N, Sucia-Foca N, Penn AS. HLA studies in patients with the Guillain-Barré syndrome. *Neurology.* 1978;28:338. Abstract.
35. Stewart JG, Pollard JD, McLeod JG, Wolnizer CM. HLA antigens in the Landry-Guillain-Barré syndrome and chronic relapsing polyneuritis. *Ann Neurol.* 1978;4:285–289.
36. McCombe PA, Clark P, Frith JA, et al. Alpha-1-antitrypsin phenotypes in demyelinating disease and the allele PiM3. *Ann Neurol.* 1985;18:514–516.
37. Feeney DJ, Pollard JD, McLeod JG, Stewart GJ, De Lange GG. Gm haplotypes in inflammatory demyelinating polyneuropathies. *Ann Neurol.* 1989;26:790–792.
38. Eiben RM, Gersony WM. Recognition, prognosis and treatment of the Guillain-Barré syndrome (acute idiopathic polyneuritis). *Med Clin North Am.* 1963;47:1294–1306.
39. Haymaker W, Kernohan JW. Landry-Guillain-Barré syndrome: clinicopathological report of 50 fatal cases and a critique of the literature. *Medicine (Baltimore).* 1949;28:59–141.
40. Loffel NB, Rossi LN, Mumenthaler M, Lutschg J, Ludin HP. The Landry-Guillain-Barré

syndrome: complications, prognosis and natural history in 123 cases. *J Neurol Sci.* 1977; 33:71–79.

41. McFarland HR, Heller GL. Guillain-Barré disease complex. *Arch Neurol.* 1966;14:196–201.
42. Melnick SC, Flewett TH. Role of infection in the Guillain-Barré syndrome. *J Neurol Neurosurg Psychiatry.* 1964;27:395–407.
43. Poser CM, Behan PO. Late onset of Guillain-Barré syndrome. *J Neuroimmunol.* 1982;3:27–41.
44. Arnason BGW. Acute inflammatory demyelinating polyradiculoneuropathies. In: Dyck PJ, Thomas PK, Lambert EH, Bunge R, eds. *Peripheral neuropathy.* Philadelphia: Saunders; 1984:2050–2100.
45. Bale JF, Rote NS, Bloomer LC, Bray PF. Guillain-Barré-like polyneuropathy after renal transplant. Possible association with cytomegalovirus infection. *Arch Neurol.* 1980;37:784.
46. Drachman DA, Paterson PY, Berlin BS, Roguska J. Immunosuppression and the Guillain-Barré syndrome. *Arch Neurol.* 1970;23:385–393.
47. Wrzolek MA, Anzil AP, Rao C, Kozlowski PB, Sher JH. Histologically proven cytomegalovirus polyradiculoneuritis in a kidney transplant recipient presenting as Guillain-Barré syndrome. *J Neuropathol Exp Neurol.* 1989;48:369. Abstract.
48. Bishopric G, Bruner J, Butler J. Guillain-Barré syndrome with cytomegalovirus infection of peripheral nerves. *Arch Pathol Lab Med.* 1985;109:1106–1108.
49. Davie CJ, Ceballos R, Little SC. Infectious mononucleosis with fatal neuronitis. *Arch Neurol.* 1963;9:265–272.
50. Eaton OM, Stevens H, Silver HM. Respiratory failure in polyradiculoneuritis associated with infectious mononucleosis. *JAMA.* 1965;194:609–611.
51. Gauthier-Smith PC. Neurological complications of glandular fever (infectious mononucleosis). *Brain.* 1965;88:323–334.
52. Raftery M, Schumaker EE, Grain GO, Quinn EL. Infectious mononucleosis and Guillain-Barré syndrome. *Arch Intern Med.* 1954;93:246–253.
53. Ricker W, Blumberg A, Peters CH, Widerman A. The association of Guillain-Barré syndrome with infectious mononucleosis with a report of 2 fatal cases. *Blood.* 1947;2:217–226.
54. Smith MS, Laguna JF. Neurological complications of infectious mononucleosis. *Pediatr Clin North Am.* 1979;26:315–326.
55. Schnell RG, Dyck PJ, Bowie EJ, Klass DW, Taswell HF. Infectious mononucleosis: neurologic and EEG findings. *Medicine (Baltimore).* 1966;45:51–65.
56. Silversides JL, Richardson JC. Neurological complications of infectious mononucleosis. *Can Med Assoc J.* 1950;63:138–143.
57. Hirano A, Cook SD, Whitaker JN, Dowling PC, Murray MR. Fine structural aspects of demyelination in vitro. The effects of Guillain-Barré serum. *J Neuropathol Exp Neurol.* 1971;30:249–265.
58. Prineas JW, Wright RG. The fine structure of peripheral nerve lesions in a virus-induced demyelinating disease in fowl (Marek's disease). *Lab Invest.* 1972;26:548–557.
59. Davies J, Rowlatt RJ. Transient severe hypertension and polyradiculitis after chicken pox. *Br Med J* 1978;2:1608–1609.
60. Welch RG. Chicken pox and the Guillain-Barré syndrome. *Arch Dis Child.* 1962;37:557–559.
61. Zivin I, Schwager VA. The Guillain-Barré syndrome as a complication of varicella. *Dis Nerve Syst.* 1972;11:742–744.
62. Dayan AD, Ogul E, Graveson GS. Polyneuritis and herpes zoster. *J Neurol Neurosurg Psychiatry.* 1972;35:170–175.
63. Hart IK, Kennedy PGE. Guillain-Barré syndrome associated with herpes zoster. *Postgrad Med J.* 1987;63:1087–1088.
64. Knox JDE, Levy R, Simpson JA. Herpes zoster and the Landry-Guillain-Barré syndrome. *J Neurol Neurosurg Psychiatry.* 1961;24:167–172.
65. Olivarius B deF, Buhl M. Herpes simplex virus and Guillain-Barré polyradiculitis. *Br Med J.* 1975;1:192–193.
66. Pepose JS. A theory of virus-induced demyelination in the Landry-Guillain-Barré syndrome. *J Neurol.* 1982;227:93–97.
67. Lane JM, Ruben FL, Neff JM, Miller JD. Complications of smallpox vaccinations. *N Engl J Med.* 1968;281:1201–1208.
68. Spillane JD, Wells CEC. Then neurology of Jennerian vaccination. *Brain.* 1964;87:1–44.
69. Cambier J, Schott B. Nosologie des polyradiculonevrites inflammatoires. *Rev Neurol.* 1966;115:811–842.

70. Parry GJ. Peripheral neuropathies associated with human immunodeficiency virus infection. *Ann Neurol.* 1988;23(suppl):549–553.
71. Cornblath DR, McArthur JC, Kennedy PGE, Witte AS, Griffin JW. Inflammatory demyelinating peripheral neuropathies associated with human T-cell lymphotrophic virus type III infection. *Ann Neurol.* 1987;21:32–40.
72. Lipkin I, Parry GJ, Kiprov D, Abrams D. Inflammatory neuropathy in homosexual men with lymphadenopathy. *Neurology.* 1985;35:1479–1483.
73. Price L, Gominak S, Raphael SA, Lischner HW, Griffin JW, Grover WD. Acute demyelinating polyneuropathy in childhood human immunodeficiency virus infection. *Ann Neurol.* 1990;28:459–460.
74. Piette AM, Tusseau F, Vignon D, et al. Acute neuropathy coincident with seroconversion for anti-LAV/HTLV-III [letter]. *Lancet.* 1986;1:852.
75. Vendrell J, Heredia C, Pujol M, Vidal J, Blesa R, Graus F. Guillain-Barré syndrome associated with seroconversion for anti-HTLV-III [letter]. *Neurology.* 1987;37:544.
76. Mishra BB, Sommers W, Koski CL, Greenstein JI. Acute inflammatory demyelinating polyneuropathy in the acquired immune deficiency syndrome. *Ann Neurol.* 1985;18:131–132. Abstract.
77. Horowitz SL, Benson DF, Gottlieb MS, Davos F, Bentson JR. Neurological complications of gay-related immunodeficiency disorder. *Ann Neurol.* 1982;12:80. Abstract.
78. Doll DC, Yarbro JW. Mycobacterial spinal abscess with an ascending polyneuropathy. *Ann Intern Med.* 1987;106:333–334.
79. Chaunu M-P, Ratinahirana H, Raphael M, et al. The spectrum of changes on 20 nerve biopsies in patients with HIV infection. *Muscle Nerve.* 1989;12:452–459.
80. Griffin JW, Cornblath DR, Becker PS, Price DL, McArthur JC. Different patterns of PNS demyelination occur in HIV infection. *J Neuropathol Exp Neurol.* 1989;48:381. Abstract.
81. Lope ES, Junquera SRC, Martinez AM, Berenguel AB. Acute ascending polyradiculoneuritis in a case of Creutzfeldt-Jakob disease. *J Neurol Neurosurg Psychiatry.* 1977;40:149–155.
82. Josiphov J, Neufeld MY, Korczyn AD. Demyelinating peripheral neuropathy in Creutzfeldt-Jakob disease (CJD). *Neurology.* 1992;42(suppl 3):268. Abstract.
83. Goldschmidt B, Menonna J, Fortunato J, Dowling P, Cook SD. Mycoplasma antibody in Guillain-Barré syndrome and other neurological disorders. *Ann Neurol.* 1980;7:108–112.
84. Steele J, Gladstone R, Thanasophon S, Fleming PC. Mycoplasma pneumonia as a determinant of the Guillain-Barré syndrome. *Lancet.* 1969;2:710–714.
85. Yesnick L. Central nervous system complications of primary atypical pneumonia. *Arch Intern Med.* 1956;97:93–97.
86. Samantray SK. Landry-Guillain-Barré-Strohl syndrome in typhoid fever. *Aust NZ J Med.* 1977;7:307–308.
87. Ropper AH. Campylobacter diarrhea and Guillain-Barré syndrome. *Arch Neurol.* 1988;45:655–656.
88. Kaldor J, Speed RB. Guillain-Barré syndrome and Campylobacter jejuni: a serological study. *Br Med J.* 1984;288:1867–1870.
89. Rhodes KM, Tattersfield AE. Guillain-Barré syndrome associated with Campylobacter infection [letter]. *Br Med J.* 1982;285:652.
90. Pryor W, Freiman JS, Gilles MA. Guillain-Barré syndrome associated with Campylobacter jejuni infection. *Aust NZ J Med.* 1984;14:687–688.
91. Speed BR, Kaldor J, Watson J. Campylobacter jejuni/Campylobacter coli-associated Guillain-Barré syndrome: immunoblot confirmation of the serological response. *Med J Aust.* 1987; 147:13–16.
92. Saida T, Kuroki S, Saida K. Guillain-Barré syndrome associated with Campylobacter jejuni infection: clinical, bacteriological and animal immunization studies. *Peripheral Nerve Study Group Abstracts.* 1991.
93. Sovilla Y, Regli F, Francioli PB. Guillain-Barré syndrome following Campylobacter jejuni enteritis. *Arch Intern Med.* 1988;148:739–741.
94. Kuroki S, Haruta T, Yoshioka M, Kobayashi Y, Nukina M, Nakanishi H. Guillain-Barré syndrome associated with Campylobacter infection. *Pediatr Infect Dis J.* 1991;10:149–151.
95. Oomes PG, van der Meche FGA, Jacobs BC, Hazenberg MP, Banffer JRJ. Antibodies to the ganglioside GM1 in sera of Guillain-Barré patients recognize epitopes on Campylobacter bacteria. *Peripheral Nerve Study Group Abstracts.* 1991.

96. van der Meche FGA, Schmitz PIM, Kleyweg RP, Meulstee J, Oomes PG. Prognostic factors in the Dutch Guillain-Barré study. *Peripheral Nerve Study Group Abstracts.* 1991.
97. Yuki N, Yoshino H, Sato S, Miyatake T. Acute axonal polyneuropathy associated with anti-GM1 antibodies following Campylobacter enteritis. *Neurology.* 1990;40:1900–1902.
98. Fujimoto S, Amako K. Guillain-Barré syndrome and Campylobacter jejuni infection [letter]. *Lancet.* 1990;335:1350.
99. Halperin JJ, Little BW, Coyle PK, Dattwyler RJ. Lyme disease: cause of a treatable peripheral neuropathy. *Neurology.* 1987;37:1700–1706.
100. Pachner AR, Steere AC. The triad of neurologic manifestations of Lyme disease: meningitis, cranial neuritis, and radiculoneuritis. *Neurology.* 1985;35:47–53.
101. Sigal LH, Tatum AH. Lyme disease patients' serum contains IgM antibodies to Borrelia burgdorferi that cross-react with neuronal antigens. *Neurology.* 1988;38:1439–1442.
102. Sterman AB, Nelson S, Barclay P. Demyelinating neuropathy accompanying Lyme disease. *Neurology.* 1982;32:1302–1305.
103. Bouma PAD, Carpay HA. Antibodies to Borrelia burgdorferi in Guillain-Barré syndrome [letter]. *Lancet.* 1989;334:739.
104. Samantray SK, Johnson SC, Mathai KV. Landry-Guillain-Barré syndrome. A study of 302 cases. *Med J Aust.* 1977;2:84–91.
105. Warembourg H, Voisin C, Furon D, Wattel F, Caron JC, Tonnel AB. Acute peripheral neuropathies associated with brucellosis. Report of 2 cases. *Lille Med.* 1969;14:536–539.
106. Melnick SC, Flewett TH. Role of infection in the Guillain-Barré syndrome. *J Neurol Neurosurg Psychiatry.* 1964;27:395–407.
107. Morgan DJR, Gawler J. Severe peripheral neuropathy complicating Legionnaire's disease. *Br Med J.* 1981;283:1577–1578.
108. Schaltenbrand G, Bammer H. La clinique et le traitement des polynevrites inflammatoires on sereuses aigues. *Rev Neurol (Paris).* 1966;115:783–810.
109. Mushinski JF, Taniguichi RM, Stiefel JW. Guillain-Barré syndrome associated with ulceroglandular tularemia. *Neurology (Minneap).* 1964;14:877–879.
110. Hemachudha T, Griffin DE, Chen WW, Johnson RT. Immunologic studies of rabies vaccination-induced Guillain-Barré syndrome. *Neurology.* 1988;38:375–378.
111. Marks JS, Halpin TJ. Guillain-Barré syndrome in recipients of A/New Jersey influenza vaccine. *JAMA.* 1980;243:2490–2494.
112. Schonberger LB, Bregman DJ, Sullivan-Bollyai JZ. Guillain-Barré syndrome following vaccination in the national influenza immunization program, United States, 1976–1977. *Am J Epidemiol.* 1979;110:105–123.
113. Hurwitz ES, Schonberger LB, Nelson DB, Holman RC. Guillain-Barré syndrome and the 1978–1979 influenza vaccine. *N Engl J Med.* 1981;304:1557–1561.
114. D'Cruz OF, Shapiro ED, Spiegelman KN, et al. Acute inflammatory demyelinating polyradiculoneuropathy (Guillain-Barré syndrome) after immunization with Haemophilus influenzae type b conjugate vaccine. *J Pediatr.* 1989;115:743–746.
115. Pollard JD, Selby G. Relapsing neuropathy due to tetanus toxoid. *J Neurol Sci.* 1978;37: 113–125.
116. Haug BA, Dressler D, Prange HW. Polyradiculoneuritis following botulinum toxin therapy. *J Neurol.* 1990;237:62–63.
117. Wiederholt WC, Mulder DW, Lambert EH. The Landry-Guillain-Barré-Strohl syndrome or polyradiculopathy: historical review, report on 97 patients and present concepts. *Mayo Clin Proc.* 1964;29:427–451.
118. Arnason BG, Asbury AK. Idiopathic polyneuritis after surgery. *Arch Neurol.* 1968;18:500–507.
119. Steiner I, Argov Z, Cahan C, Abramsky O. Guillain-Barré syndrome after epidural anesthesia: direct nerve root damage may trigger disease. *Neurology.* 1985;35:1473–1475.
120. Parry GJ, Heiman-Patterson TD. Pregnancy and autoimmune neuromuscular disease. *Semin Neurol.* 1988;8:197–204.
121. Asbury AK, Arnason BG, Adams RD. The inflammatory lesion in idiopathic polyneuritis. *Medicine (Baltimore).* 1969;48:173–215.
122. Julien J, Vital CL, Aupy G, Lagueny A, Darriet D, Brechenmacher C. Guillain-Barré syndrome and Hodgkins disease—ultrastructural study of peripheral nerve. *J Neurol Sci.* 1980;45:23–27.
123. Klingon GH. The Guillain-Barré syndrome associated with cancer. *Cancer.* 1965;18:157–163.
124. Lisak RP, Mitchell M, Zweiman B, Orrechio E, Asbury AK. Guillain-Barré syndrome and Hodgkins disease: three cases with immunological studies. *Ann Neurol.* 1977;1:72–78.

125. Strickland GT, Moser KM. Sarcoidosis with a Landry-Guillain-Barré syndrome and clinical response to corticosteroids. *Am J Med*. 1967;43:131–135.
126. Miller R, Sheron N, Semple S. Sarcoidosis presenting with an acute Guillain-Barré syndrome. *Postgrad Med J*. 1989;65:765–767.
127. Godwin JE, Sahn SA. Sarcoidosis presenting as progressive ascending lower extremity weakness and asymptomatic meningitis with hypoglycorrhachia. *Chest*. 1990;97:1263–1265.
128. Valbonesi M, Mosconi L, Garelli S, Zerbi D, Celano I. Successful treatment by plasma exchange in Guillain-Barré syndrome with immune complexes. *Vox Sang*. 1980;38:181–184.
129. Behan PO, Stilmant M, Lowenstein LM, Sax DS. Landry-Guillain-Barré-Strohl syndrome and immune-complex nephritis. *Lancet*. 1973;1:850–854.
130. Chaudhuri KR, Taylor IK, Niven RM, Abbott RJ. A case of systemic lupus erythematosis presenting as Guillain-Barré syndrome. *Br J Rheumatol*. 1989;28:440–442.
131. Frederick WG, Enriquez R, Bookbinder MJ. Peripheral neuropathy associated with $_1$-antitrypsin deficiency. *Arch Neurol*. 1990;47:233–235.
132. Katrak SM, Pollock M, O'Brien CP, et al. Clinical and morphological features of gold neuropathy. *Brain*. 1980;103:671–693.
133. Dick DJ, Raman D. The Guillain-Barré syndrome following gold therapy. *Scand J Rheumatol*. 1982;11:119–120.
134. Roquer J, Herraiz J, Maymo J, Olive A, Carbonell J. Miller-Fisher syndrome (Guillain-Barré syndrome with ophthalmoplegia) during treatment with gold salts in a patient with rheumatoid arthritis. *Arthritis Rheum*. 1985;28:838–839.
135. Knezevic W, Quintner J, Mastaglia FL, Zilko PJ. Guillain-Barré syndrome and pemphigus foliaceus associated with D-penicillamine therapy. *Aust NZ J Med*. 1984;14:50–52.
136. Regev I, Bornstein N, Carasso R, Vardi Y. Acute polyneuropathy combined with myasthenia gravis. *Acta Neurol Scand*. 1982;65:681–682.
137. Carlander B, Touchon J, Georgesco M, Cadilhac J. Myasthenia gravis and recurrent Guillain-Barré syndrome. *Neurology*. 1991;41:1848.
138. Eden KV. Possible association of Guillain-Barré syndrome with thrombolytic therapy [letter]. *JAMA*. 1983;249:2020–2021.
139. Leaf DA, McDonald I, Kliks B, Willison R, Jones SR. Streptokinase and the Guillain-Barré syndrome [letter]. *Ann Intern Med*. 1984;100:617.
140. Arrowsmith JB, Milstein JB, Kuritsky JN, Murano G. Streptokinase and the Guillain-Barré syndrome [letter]. *Ann Intern Med*. 1985;103:302.
141. Cicale MJ. Guillain-Barré after streptokinase therapy [letter]. *South Med J*. 1987;80:1068.
142. Roquer J, Herraiz D, Arnau R, Serrat. Guillain-Barré syndrome after streptokinase therapy [letter]. *Acta Neurol Scand*. 1990;82:153.
143. Atkinson AB, Brown JJ, Lever AF, et al. Neurological dysfunction in two patients receiving captopril and cimetidine. *Lancet*. 1980;2:36–37.
144. Chakraborty TK, Ruddell WSJ. Guillain-Barré neuropathy during treatment with captopril. *Postgrad Med J*. 1987;63:221–222.
145. Hory B, Blanc D, Boillot A, Panouse-Perrin J. Guillain-Barré syndrome following danazol and corticosteroid therapy for hereditary angioedema. *Am J Med*. 1985;79:111–114.
146. Fagius J, Osterman PO, Siden A, Wiholm B-E. Guillain-Barré syndrome following zimeldine treatment. *J Neurol Neurosurg Psychiatry*. 1985;48:65–69.
147. Leys D, Pasquier F, Lamblin MD, Dubois F, Petit H. Acute polyradiculoneuropathy after amitriptyline overdose. *Br Med J*. 1987;294:608.
148. Loizou LA, Boddie HG. Polyradiculoneuropathy associated with heroin abuse. *J Neurol Neurosurg Psychiatry*. 1978;41:855–857.
149. Richter RW, Pearson J, Bruun B, Challenor YB, Brust JCM, Baden MM. Neurological complications of addiction to heroin. *Bull NY Acad Med*. 1973;49:3–21.
150. Smith WR, Wilson AF. Guillain-Barré syndrome in heroin addiction. *JAMA*. 1975;231:1367–1368.

8

Pathology

Although symptoms of neuropathy had been long recognized, the first description of the pathological changes in neuropathy did not appear until 1864 when Dumenil[1] described the pathology in the nerves of a patient who died from a subacutely progressive, ascending paralysis with distal sensory loss. There was loss of nerve fibers in the distal peripheral nerves of the arms and legs but the nerve roots as well as the spinal cord and brain were normal. Probably the first descriptions of the pathology of Guillain-Barré syndrome (GBS) were those of Dejerine and Goetz[2] and of Westfall,[3] both in 1876; other reports soon followed.[4,5] These earliest reports noted that the peripheral nerve changes were predominantly proximal in distribution, an observation that has been repeatedly confirmed. The presence of inflammation in some cases was recognized shortly thereafter.[6,7] Inflammatory cells, predominantly lymphocytes, were noted to be less frequent early in the course of the paralysis, leading to the suggestion that they were present as a response to nerve injury rather than as an integral part of the initial pathological process.[8] The predominantly demyelinating nature of the pathology was also recognized early but not emphasized, and its significance was not appreciated until the discovery of experimental allergic neuritis by Waksman and Adams in 1955.[9] The quintessential pathological features of the disease are now considered to be macrophage-mediated demyelination accompanied by inflammation.

Macroscopic Abnormalities

The peripheral nerves, including the roots, are usually normal macroscopically. Swelling has been reported on occasion[8,10,11] but is an inconstant feature. Haymaker and Kernohan[8] noted that edema of nerves was seen in patients dying in the first week of illness, sometimes as the only significant abnormality. They also found that edema was sometimes present at later stages and was prominent in one case of 46 days' duration. By contrast, Asbury et al.[12] and Arnason[13] failed to find any macroscopic evidence of nerve swelling in any of their cases. Microscopic edema, concentrated in the subperineurial space and extending along the intrafascicular septae, may be seen, even when the nerve is not overtly swollen.

Inflammatory Changes

The presence of chronic inflammatory cells, predominantly lymphocytes, is considered by some to be the hallmark of this disease.[12] They are found scattered throughout the peripheral nervous system, including the nerve roots, plexuses, and nerve trunks. They are also seen, and may be prominent, in the dorsal root ganglia,[8,12] sympathetic chains and ganglia,[14] and intramuscular arborization of motor nerves, all the way to the finest myelinated motor nerve branches.[12] Mononuclear cells have even been seen within axons in ultrastructural studies.[15] In one study they were not found in cutaneous nerve branches even though there was severe myelin degeneration, perhaps because the loss of myelin was secondary to wallerian degeneration from more proximally placed inflammatory lesions.[16] Lymphocytes may be seen in the endoneurium, scattered diffusely between nerve bundles or in both the endoneurium and epineurium, concentrated around small blood vessels, particularly venules. The intensity of the inflammatory response varies enormously; in some cases it is confined to a few scattered perivascular lymphocytes whereas in others, sheets of lymphocytes are seen almost obliterating the architecture of the underlying nerve (Fig. 8–1). Early in the disease, particularly with intensely destructive lesions, a few polymorphonuclear leukocytes may be seen admixed with the lymphocytes; later, plasma cells appear. Several authors have noted a paucity of inflammation in the nerves of patients dying within a few days of the onset of symptoms.[8,17] For example, Haymaker and Kernohan[8] examined the nerves of 22 patients who died within a week of the onset of symptoms and found no inflammation; the only abnormality noted was nerve edema and early fragmentation of the myelin and axons. Small collections of lymphocytes appeared during the second week and increased thereafter. They concluded that the lymphocytes represented a part of the reparative process and played no role in the pathogenesis of the disease. Asbury et al.[12] disputed these observations. In their group of 19 cases, the 4 who died early, within the first week of illness, all had well developed inflammatory changes without gross or microscopic edema. Furthermore, they noted that myelin destruction was confined to those regions of the peripheral nerves that were infiltrated with inflammatory cells. They concluded that inflammation preceded or coincided with the clinical onset and ascribed a critical pathogenetic role to lymphocytes in the process of demyelination. Others have also noted inflammation in patients dying during the first week.[18–20]

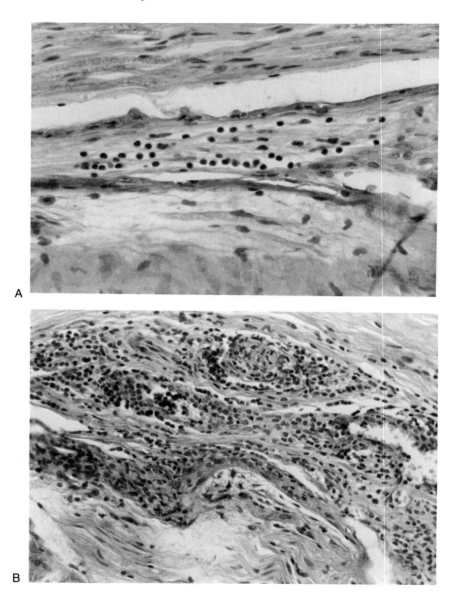

A

B

Figure 8–1. Inflammatory changes in GBS vary enormously and may be completely absent. In some cases inflammation is confined to a few scattered lymphocytes, concentrated around epineurial vessels (**A**) or there may be intense, diffuse inflammation as shown in the lower panel (**B**).

The findings in autopsy studies may not be representative of all cases of GBS, especially those patients who die early, since they represent the most severe end of the spectrum of the disease. Biopsy studies may therefore give information more applicable to typical disease. Conversely, the disadvantage of biopsy studies is that sensory nerves such as the sural nerve are not the primary site of involvement in GBS and pathological changes seen there may not accurately reflect the pathology at other, more involved sites such as the nerve root. With that caveat in mind, there are significant differences in the nerve pathology in biopsy specimens, particularly with regard to the presence of inflammatory cells. Brechenmacher et al.[15] found that mononuclear cells were present by light microscopy in only 5 out of 57 biopsy specimens. Julien et al.[21] examined a sural nerve biopsy from a single patient with GBS that developed during remission from Hodgkin's disease. There was no evidence of lymphocytic infiltration; rather, macrophages were seen invading and phagocytosing normal myelin. In contrast, Prineas[22] examined biopsy material from nine GBS patients and found macrophage-mediated demyelination in six, always in association with infiltrating lymphocytes. Lymphocytes were present in both early and late cases, even in a patient biopsied within 2 days of the onset of symptoms. However, more intense lymphocytic infiltration was seen in patients biopsied 1 week or more into the disease. Honavar et al.[23] and Hughes et al.,[24] in further biopsy studies, found that macrophage-mediated demyelination was common and proceeded in the absence of lymphocytic infiltration. Inflammatory cells were rarely seen, except in patients with human immunodeficiency virus (HIV) infection. They suggested that the pathology and the pathogenesis of the demyelination are heterogeneous, with some cases being mediated by a cellular mechanism and others by circulating (humoral) antibodies with demyelination in the latter proceeding in the absence of lymphocytes. Additional indirect evidence that lymphocytes may not play a central role in the progression of demyelination comes from a study by Feasby.[25] Very early in the course of the disease, he treated GBS patients with anti–T cell monoclonal antibodies. Although the patients developed acute lymphopenia, there was continued progression of the clinical deficit for several days, suggesting that lymphocytes are not essential for the progression of demyelination, although these observations do not exclude a role in its initiation. Thus, the concept that lymphocytes play a central role in the pathogenesis of demyelination in GBS remains controversial.

Central to this controversy about the timing of the appearance of inflammatory cells is the argument concerning the respective roles of cell-mediated and humoral immunity in the pathogenesis of GBS, an argument that is developed further in Chapter 9. Arnason[13] argues that the pathological lesions, from the morphologic standpoint, are in every way typical of a delayed hypersensitivity reaction whereas Hughes et al.[24] suggest that the immunopathological reaction is not stereotyped and that cellular and humoral mechanisms may be operating in different cases. In cases in which there is early infiltration of lymphocytes, preceding or accompanying the destruction of myelin by macrophages, the basic immunological mechanism is perhaps more likely to be cell-mediated autoimmunity and the disease analogous to EAN. When the pathology is characterized by early dissolution and vesiculation of normal myelin accompanied by phagocytosis, particularly in those cases in which this process proceeds in the absence of lymphocytic infiltration, the pathogenesis of the demyelination is more likely to be humorally mediated, perhaps analogous to the demyelination induced by intraneural injection of antibodies to galactocerebroside. Although no specific humoral antibody to myelin has been consistently demonstrated in GBS, the response to plasmapheresis and the ability of serum from patients to demyelinate nerve when it is introduced directly into the endoneurial compartment of recipient animals also suggest a role for circulating antibodies in the pathogenesis of the demyelination.

A curious feature noted by many is the persistence of inflammation in this monophasic disease, whose clinical course reaches a nadir within 3 to 4 weeks and is usually followed by uninterrupted recovery and only rarely relapses. Some of the cases described by Asbury et al.[12] survived for several weeks; in these patients, areas of both recent and remote inflammatory demyelination were found, suggesting that the inflammatory processing was ongoing, even though the clinical course was monophasic. In other cases, a low grade inflammatory process persisted for months and even years. Similarly, the longest surviving patient of Haymaker and Kernohan,[8] who survived for 46 days, still showed inflammation; others have also noted persistent inflammation in patients dying up to 17 weeks after the onset of disease. It is possible that a proportion of these patients were really suffering from chronic inflammatory demyelinating polyradiculoneuropathy, which had an acute presentation but this is an unlikely explanation for most cases. The significance of these persistent inflammatory changes remains unclear.

Myelin and Schwann Cell Changes

Demyelination

Degeneration of myelin was recognized early as a constant feature of GBS. However, early reports did not make a clear distinction between primary and secondary demyelination. For example, Haymaker and Kernohan,[8] although recognizing the early swelling and irregularity of the myelin sheath that occurred in the first few days, gave equal cognizance to disintegration of the axons. In fact, in their series there was an unusually striking degree of axonal degeneration, probably reflecting the severity of these fatal cases since this was an autopsy series. However, even in the biopsy case reported by Finean and Woolf,[16] axonal degeneration was prominent, at least in cutaneous nerves, and was felt to represent the primary pathology. Segmental demyelination was not established as the primary pathology until 1969, when the careful pathological studies of Wisniewski et al.[26] and Asbury et al.[12] were reported. In their ultrastructural study of a single fatal case, dying 14 days after the onset of weakness, Wisniewski et al. clearly demonstrated macrophage stripping of ultrastructurally normal myelin away from the underlying axons, as shown in Figures 8–2 and 8–3. Similarly, the detailed light microscopic study of Asbury et al. showed that the predominant abnormality was segmental demyelination, which they found to be restricted to areas of nerve corresponding to infiltration of lymphocytes. However, axonal degeneration was also seen frequently, particularly in areas of intense inflammation. Prineas,[22] in a study of sural nerve biopsies, found that demyelination was more randomly distributed and had no particular relationship to foci of inflammatory cells or to blood vessels. Not surprisingly, in this biopsy series of less severely involved cases, there was less axonal degeneration.

Subsequent detailed ultrastructural studies reported by Prineas[27] and others[28–30] have established the primary nature of the demyelination and the sequence of events. There have been a few reports of vesiculation of myelin and splitting of myelin lamellae, in the absence of cellular infiltration, as the earliest change (Fig. 8–4). These findings were initially reported in autopsy specimens and may have been, at least in some cases, autolytic artifact. However, Wisniewski et al.[26] found similar vesicular changes in the nerves from their patient, which were always associated with macrophages if serial or reorientated sections were examined, suggesting that they were not artifactual. Vesiculation of myelin has also been seen in biopsy specimens[22,27,31,32] in which artifact due to poor fixation is less likely. The vesicles are formed by separation of adjacent myelin lamellae, along the major dense line.[15,29] They may appear as both round and elongated profiles, suggesting that they have a tubular shape. Similar vesicular disruption of myelin constitutes the earliest abnormality seen in the studies of experimental demyelination, induced by intraneural injection of either galactocerebroside antibodies[33] or human GBS serum,[34,35] models of humorally induced demyelination. The similarity between the vesiculation of myelin seen in early GBS and in the models of experimental demyelination helps to fuel the controversy concerning the respective roles of cell-mediated and humoral immunity in the pathogenesis of the demyelination. Some investigators have argued that the primary pathological change is antibody-induced myelin vesiculation, perhaps accentuated at sites where the blood–nerve barrier is relatively deficient or where it has been damaged, enabling circulating antibodies to gain access to the endoneurial space and bind to myelin.[33,36,37] Following this line of reasoning, the associated macrophage-mediated myelin stripping and lymphocytic infiltration represent a reactive change. This could explain why inflammation is sparse or completely lacking in some of the earliest cases.

The next change seen, more prominently in the vicinity of the lymphocytic infiltrates if they are present, is penetration of macrophages through the basal lamina of the Schwann cell[13] (Figs. 8–2 and 8–3). The Schwann cell

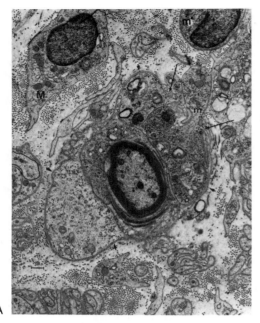

A

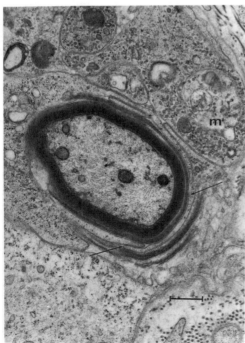

B

Figure 8–2. Most often, demyelination is a macrophage-initiated process as shown in this biopsy of a patient with early GBS. In **A**, a macrophage process (*m*) has insinuated itself through the Schwann cell basal lamina (*long arrows*) and can be seen separating the outer few lamellae from the underlying myelin sheath. The remainder of the basal lamina, indicated by the short arrows, is undisturbed. A mononuclear cell lies close by (*M*) and another macrophage (*m'*) lies above and to the right. **B** is a higher power electron photomicrograph of the same axon. A long macrophage process (*arrows*) can be seen stripping away the outer myelin lamellae. (Photomicrographs provided by Dr. John Pollard.)

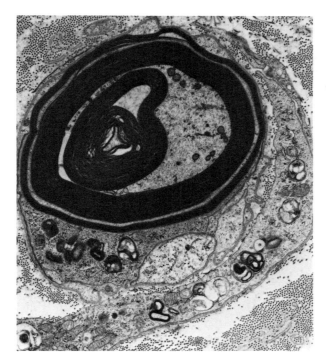

Figure 8–3. Although myelin stripping most often involves the outer lamellae, adaxonal myelin may also be affected early. In this electron photomicrograph, a macrophage process can be seen separating the outer myelin lamellae but the adaxonal lamellae are also compromised. (Photomicrograph provided by Dr. John Pollard.)

cytoplasm is displaced away from the adjacent myelin sheath, which may still appear ultrastructurally normal. Macrophages then insinuate organelle-free processes between the myelin lamellae, along the interperiod lines, and groups of intact myelin lamellae are phagocytosed. Macrophage processes may even extend down to the adaxonal space (Fig. 8–3) and have been described within myelinated axons, perhaps accounting for some of the associated axonal degeneration.[15] In the case described by Wisniewski et al.,[26] there was no particular relationship between the node of Ranvier and invading macrophages. However, others[29] have noted that the earliest change is retraction of the terminal myelin loops from the node of Ranvier causing widening of the nodal gap, followed by paranodal myelin degeneration, which proceeds centripetally toward the Schwann cell nucleus. In addition, there may be a predilection for early involvement at the Schmidt-Lanterman incisure. This distribution of pathological changes is similar to those seen in antiserum-induced demyelination in experimental animals. This earliest pathological change in the paranodal apparatus would result in a marked increase in capacitance of the nodal axolemma, leading to conduction block,

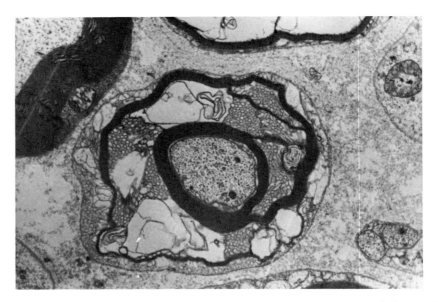

Figure 8–4.   Vesiculation of myelin of the type seen in this Figure may occasionally be seen in GBS, in the absence of mononuclear cell infiltration. The tubular aggregates can be clearly seen. The Schwann cell basement membrane is intact and no macrophage stripping has yet occurred.

even when the pathological changes of demyelination are apparently trivial. This explains the relative paucity of pathological changes despite severe paralysis in some patients who die in the first few days of the illness. Ultimately, there is complete demyelination (Fig. 8–5), usually involving several adjacent internodes.

Remyelination

There is a remarkable paucity of information concerning the process of remyelination in GBS. Equally remarkable is the paucity of remyelination seen in patients whose nervous tissue has been harvested as much as 7 weeks after the onset of symptoms. Prineas[22] found little evidence of remyelination in sural nerve biopsies from nine patients with GBS whose duration of disease ranged from 2 to 49 days. Examination of one patient, who died 50 days after onset of disease, revealed that most axons in nerve roots were invested with only a few myelin lamellae whereas others were still entirely denuded. Changes in nerves at other locations were not described. Liu[38] described vesicular changes in the myelin during the clinical recovery phase of a patient who died 17 days after onset. He attributed this vesiculation to remyelination, suggesting that the vesicles coalesced to form new myelin. However, even though the patient had begun to recover clinically, these

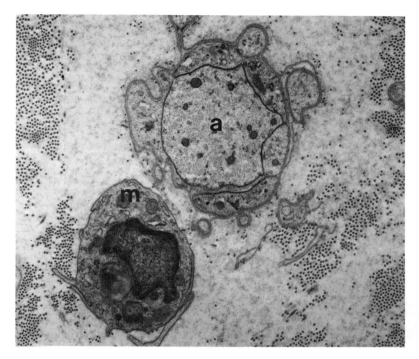

Figure 8–5. In this electron photomicrograph of more advanced demyelination in GBS, a completely demyelinated axon (*a*) is seen lying alongside a mononuclear cell (*m*). (Photomicrograph provided by Dr. John Pollard.)

pathological findings are more likely to represent ongoing myelin degeneration. Several other autopsy studies of patients dying between 1 and 3 weeks after the onset of neurological symptoms have noted no evidence of remyelination, leading to the suggestion that remyelination might be inhibited while active disease persists.[27] However, Vital and Vallat[39] have noted the coexistence of demyelinating and remyelinating axons within the same fascicle, although they do not note the time at which the specimens were obtained in relationship to the onset of symptoms. There is clinical recovery, beginning within the first week or two in some nerves, even while other areas are deteriorating; the electrophysiological studies in humans[40,41] and experimental animals[42] indicate that recovery is most likely being brought about by remyelination, resulting in reversal of conduction block. Therefore, it is most likely that the infrequency with which remyelination is seen in pathological specimens is primarily a result of sampling, at least in the biopsy studies. Since the autopsied cases are the most severe ones it is possible that, in these patients, there is remyelination inhibition.

Although there are few studies of remyelination in GBS, the pattern and sequence of remyelination can be implied by analogy with chronic relapsing demyelinating neuropathy as well as with experimental demyelinating neuropathies. In the former, after the macrophages leave, cytoplasmic extensions of the original Schwann cell reinvest the underlying demyelinated axon but do not participate in its remyelination.[43,44] Eventually, they are replaced with Schwann cells of a different appearance, rich in granular endoplasmic reticulum and with many polyribosomes, which carry out the remyelination.[39] After experimental demyelination in rats, induced by intraneural injection of antibodies to galactocerebroside, the earliest evidence of remyelination is seen about 8 days after antibody injection.[42] At this time, some axons are surrounded by a few turns of compacted myelin whereas others are invested with uncompacted myelin. Most axons were still demyelinated. Thereafter, there was a progressive increase in the number of axons myelinating, without apparent relationship to axon diameter, as well as increasing thickness of myelin around each axon and compaction of the lamellae. By extrapolation to the clinical situation, remyelination would not be expected in tissue harvested during the first week after the onset of symptoms but should progressively increase thereafter. Although myelin thickness increases with time it may never achieve the full thickness of original myelin. Because the myelin remains thinner and because there are more nodes of Ranvier, some conduction slowing may last indefinitely after recovery from GBS and some tendon reflexes may fail to return.

Schwann Cell Changes

Although Schwann cells are probably capable of participating in the phagocytosis of myelin, they do not appear to do so in GBS to any significant extent, although they occasionally are seen containing myelin debris. Those Schwann cells whose myelin has been destroyed do not appear normal, showing depletion and dilatation of the rough endoplasmic reticulum and sparse, watery cytoplasm.[29] They do not participate in the brisk Schwann cell proliferation, which begins about a week after the onset of symptoms, nor in the subsequent remyelination. Rather, they are displaced by proliferating Schwann cells perhaps derived from adjacent unaffected nerve segments or from pluripotential endoneurial stem cells, which migrate into the area of demyelination. Although the exact derivation of the proliferating Schwann cells is obscure, Schwann cells from normally myelinated internodes have been seen extending thin cytoplasmic tentacles into the adjacent demyelinated segments, suggesting that undamaged Schwann cells are at least capable of participating in the remyelination process. As proliferating Schwann cells migrate into demyelinated segments of nerve, the territory of a single original Schwann cell is taken over and remyelinated by several new Schwann cells. As a result, new internodes are shorter and there is marked variation in internodal length. In addition, there are more nodes of Ranvier. Examination of single teased myelinated fibers shows that internodal length and myelin thickness both vary. Schwann cells proliferate more vigorously in areas of wallerian degeneration and align themselves in longitudinal rows within the basement membrane (bands of Bungner) as a prelude to regeneration.

Axonal Changes

Although GBS is a primarily demyelinating neuropathy, there is almost invariably some degree of associated axonal degeneration. In addition, there are changes in the appearance of axons underlying areas of demyelination. In the early autopsy studies of Haymaker and Kernohan[8] and of Asbury et al.[12] there was a striking amount of wallerian degeneration, presumably reflecting the severity of these cases that lead to death. However, even biopsy of a cutaneous nerve from a patient with nonfatal disease showed changes of wallerian degeneration as the only significant abnormality.[16] This is not altogether surprising since cutaneous nerve does not bear the brunt of demyelination and any changes seen probably reflect only axonal damage at more proximal levels. More recently, Feasby et al.[45] studied a group of patients with acute areflexic paralysis that fit all the National Institute of Neurological and Communicative Disorders and Stroke (NINCDS) criteria for GBS and yet their primary electrophysiological abnormalities indicated axonal degeneration. One patient was examined at autopsy; there was severe and widespread axonal degeneration with some clusters of regenerating axons but no evidence of segmental demyelination. Vallat et al.[46] have also described GBS patients with severe axonal degeneration but their cases, unlike that of Feasby et al., also had associated demyelination. Yuki et al.[47] reported two cases of GBS after *Campylobacter jejuni* enteritis and associated with antibodies to GM1 ganglioside, in whom axonal degeneration was particularly prominent. They suggested that the anti-GM1 antibodies might be involved in the pathogenesis of the axonal degeneration, although an equally plausible explanation is that the anti-GM1 antibodies were produced in response to severe axonal degeneration. From these studies it is clear that axonal degeneration can be a prominent feature of GBS and it carries an ominous prognosis. However, even in milder cases there is some evidence of axonal degeneration, particularly in regions of intense inflammation.

Axonal changes, without overt degeneration, are also seen in demyelinated nerve segments. The axon diameter is reduced, sometimes as much as 50%, and the neurofilaments, neurotubules, and other intraaxonal organelles are more densely packed.[27] Occasionally axonal changes have been described, occurring without specific relationship to myelin or Schwann cell abnormalities. These changes occur primarily in the region of the node of Ranvier and consist of protrusion of nodal axoplasm into the nodal gap and into the paranodal periaxonal space. The significance of such changes is unclear but they may represent response to axonal injury at a slightly more distal level. In most studies, unmyelinated axons are normal although they are occasionally reduced in number.[39]

Central Nervous System Changes

The earliest reports of the pathology in GBS gave undue emphasis to the central nervous system (CNS) changes. Many of the reported abnormalities were in tissue taken from patients with a protracted course in whom the pathology was almost certainly unrelated to the primary pathological process. The most common change is central chromatolysis of anterior horn motor neurons and the motor cranial nerve nuclei, secondary to wallerian degeneration of peripheral axons. This reactive change is seen most prominently in severe cases. Similarly, degeneration of posterior column axons may be seen in cases in which there is severe dorsal root or dorsal root ganglion involvement. Very rarely, in severe cases there may be small collections of perivascular lymphocytes in the spinal cord. Somewhat more frequent, but still rare, is mild lymphocytic infiltration of the leptomeninges, which may explain the sometime presence of CSF pleocytosis. Primary changes in CNS myelin, analogous to those seen peripherally, have not been reported. In those rare cases that have been described with optic neuritis, there is presumably inflammatory demyelination of the optic nerve but pathological studies have not been reported.

Distribution of Lesions and Temporal Sequence

Most studies have emphasized that the lesions in GBS are located primarily proximally, particularly in ventral nerve roots or where the ventral and dorsal roots fuse to form the spinal nerve. However, Arnason[13] noted that foci of inflammation, with associated myelin breakdown, were scattered throughout the peripheral nervous system without any particular predilection for nerve roots in general or the ventral roots in particular. He felt that the emphasis on nerve roots in earlier reports was because nerve roots were more frequently available for pathological examination since they were removed along with the spinal cord. Nonetheless, the accentuation of involvement in nerve roots, particularly in the early stages of the disease, accords with both the electrophysiological findings and the almost invariable elevation of CSF protein. In fact, in occasional mild cases, demyelination seems to be confined to ventral roots by electrophysiological criteria. In most cases, as the disease progresses, inflammatory demyelinating lesions appear at every level of peripheral nerves including the most distal myelinated motor nerve twigs, just proximal to the neuromuscular junction, and myelinated sympathetic nerves. There may also be inflammatory lesions in the dorsal root and sympathetic ganglia. Sequential nerve conduction studies in GBS suggest that there is early and preferential involvement of the most distal, intramuscular motor nerve twigs and at sites of nerve trunks prone to compression such as the carpal tunnel and the cubital tunnel as well as ventral nerve roots. Common to each of these sites is a relative deficiency of the normal blood–

nerve barrier. This suggests that they may be sites at which a circulating humoral antibody could preferentially gain access to the endoneurial space and hence to myelin and provides further circumstantial evidence that humoral mechanisms may be important in the pathogenesis of the demyelination in GBS. However, there are no pathological studies to support these physiological observations.

The temporal sequence of pathological events has been established in many studies of fatal cases but is not known with certainty in mild disease. There is a remarkable paucity of abnormalities in those patients who die within the first week. Haymaker and Kernohan[8] emphasized the presence of edema as the earliest change seen in a patient who died at 4 days, but Asbury et al.[12] disputed this. Between days 5 and 7 there is increasing irregularity in myelin sheaths seen by light microscopy, which translates into loosening and vesiculation of myelin, particularly at nodes of Ranvier and Schmidt-Lanterman incisures, when viewed with the electron microscope. During this first week many reports have noted that inflammation is less prominent or, in some cases, even absent. Some time during the second week there is the beginning of remyelination, although in severe cases this may be delayed. Recovery of function appears to parallel the stage of remyelination.

Summary

The primary pathological lesion in GBS is macrophage-mediated demyelination, the brunt of which is borne by nerve roots. There is controversy regarding the respective roles of cell-mediated and humoral immunity in the pathogenesis of the demyelination but the bulk of the evidence favors a primary role for the former. Some axonal degeneration is seen and may be severe. Recovery takes place by means of remyelination, which begins within a few weeks and proceeds over several months.

References

1. Dumenil L. Paralysie peripherique du mouvement et du sentiment portant sur les quartres membres. Atrophie des rameaux nerveux des parties paralysees. *Gaz Hebdom Med*. 1864; 1:203–207.
2. Dejerine J, Goetz A. Note sur un cas de paralysie ascendante aigue. *Arch Physiol*. 1876;8:312–322.
3. Westfall C. Uber einege Falle von acuter todtlicher spinallahmung (sogenannter acuter aufsteigender Paralyse). *Arch Psychiatry*. 1876;6:765–822.
4. Eichhorst H. Neuritis acuta progressiva. *Virch Arch Pathol Anat*. 1877;69:265–274.
5. Mills CK. The reclassification of some organic nervous diseases on the basis of the neuron. *JAMA*. 1898;31:11–13. Abstract.
6. Thomas JJ. Two cases of acute ascending paralysis, with autopsy. *Am J Med Sci*. 1898;116: 113–148.
7. Boinet J. Un cas de paralysie de Landry. *Gaz Hop*. 1899;22:468–476.
8. Haymaker W, Kernohan JW. The Landry-Guillain-Barré syndrome. A clinicopathological report of fifty fatal cases and a critique of the literature. *Medicine*. 1949;28:59–141.
9. Waksman BH, Adams RA. Allergic neuritis: an experimental disease of rabbits induced by the injection of peripheral nervous tissue and adjuvants. *J Exp Med*. 1955;102:213–235.

10. Scheinker M. Pathology and pathogenesis of infectious polyneuritis. *Trans Am Neurol Assoc.* 1947;72:141–142.
11. Krucke W. Die primar-entzundliche polyneuritis unbekannter ursache. In: Lubarsch O, Henke F, Rossle G, eds. *Handbuch der speziellen pathologischen anatomie und histologie. Vol 13, Erkrankungen der peripheren nerven.* Berlin: Springer; 1955:164–182.
12. Asbury AK, Arnason GB, Adams RD. The inflammatory lesion in idiopathic polyneuritis. Its role in pathogenesis. *Medicine.* 1969;48:173–215.
13. Arnason BG. Acute inflammatory demyelinating polyradiculoneuropathies. In: Dyck PJ, Thomas PK, Lambert EH, Bunge R, eds. *Peripheral neuropathy.* Philadelphia: Saunders; 1984: 2050–2100.
14. Matsuyama H, Haymaker W. Distribution of lesions in the Landry-Guillain-Barré syndrome, with emphasis on involvement of the sympathetic system. *Acta Neuropathol.* 1967;8:230–241.
15. Brechenmacher C, Vital C, Laurentjoye L, Castaigne Y. Ultrastructural study of peripheral nerve in Guillain-Barré syndrome. Presence of mononuclear cells in axons. *Acta Neuropathol.* 1981;7(suppl):249–251.
16. Finean JB, Woolf AL. An electron microscope study of degenerative changes in human cutaneous nerve. *J Neuropathol Exp Neurol.* 1962;21:105–115.
17. Kanda T, Hayashi H, Tanabe H, Tsubaki T, Oda M. A fulminant case of Guillain-Barré syndrome: topographic and fibre size related analysis of demyelinating changes. *J Neurol Neurosurg Psychiatry.* 1989;52:857–864.
18. Pette H, Kornyey S. Zur histologie und pathogeneseder akut-entzundlichen formen der Landryschen paralyse. *Ztschr Neurol Psychiatry.* 1930;128:390–398.
19. Demme H. Zur pathogenese der entzundlichen formen der Landryschen paralyse. *Dtsch Ztschr Nervenh.* 1932;125:1–17.
20. Aring CD. Infectious polyneuritis. *Int Clin.* 1945;4:262–274.
21. Julien J, Vital C, Aupy G, Lagueny A, Darriet D, Brechenmacher C. Guillain-Barré syndrome and Hodgkin's disease. Ultrastructural study of a peripheral nerve. *J Neurol Sci.* 1980;45:23–27.
22. Prineas JW. Acute idiopathic polyneuritis. An electron microscopic study. *Lab Invest.* 1972; 26:133–147.
23. Honavar M, Tharakan JKJ, Hughes RAC, Leibowitz, Winer JB. A clinicopathological study of the Guillain-Barré syndrome: nine cases and a literature review. *Brain.* 1991;114:1245–1269.
24. Hughes R, Atkinson P, Coates P, Hall S, Leibowitz S. Sural nerve biopsies in Guillain-Barré syndrome: axonal degeneration and macrophage-associated demyelination and absence of cytomegalovirus genome. *Muscle Nerve.* 1992;15:568–575.
25. Feasby T. Treatment of Guillain-Barré syndrome with anti-T cell monoclonal antibodies. *J Neurol Neurosurg Psychiatry.* 1991;54:51–54.
26. Wisniewski H, Terry RD, Whitaker JN, Cook SD, Dowling PC. Landry-Guillain-Barré syndrome. A primary demyelinating disease. *Arch Neurol.* 1969;21:269–276.
27. Prineas JW. Pathology of the Guillain-Barré syndrome. *Ann Neurol.* 1981;9(suppl):6–19.
28. Hart MN, Hanks DT, Mackay R. Ultrastructural observations in Guillain-Barré syndrome. *Arch Pathol.* 1972;93:552–555.
29. Carpenter S. An ultrastructural study of an acute fatal case of the Guillain-Barré syndrome. *J Neurol Sci.* 1972;15:125–140.
30. Arstila AU, Riekkinen PJ, Rinne UK, Pelliniemi TT, Nevalainen T. Guillain-Barré syndrome. Neurochemical and ultrastructural study. *Eur Neurol.* 1971;5:257–269.
31. Miyakawa T, Murayama E, Sumiyoshi S, et al. A biopsy case of Landry-Guillain-Barré syndrome. *Acta Neuropathol.* 1971;17:181–187.
32. Brechenmacher C, Vital C, Deminiere C, et al. Guillain-Barré syndrome: an ultrastructural study of peripheral nerve in 65 patients. *Clin Neuropathol.* 1987;6:19–24.
33. Saida K, Saida T, Brown MJ, Silberberg DH, Asbury AK. Antiserum-mediated demyelination in vivo. A sequential study using intraneural injection of experimental allergic neuritis serum. *Lab Invest.* 1978;39:449–462.
34. Saida, T, Saida K, Lisak RP, Brown MJ, Silberberg DH, Asbury AK. In vivo demyelinating activity of sera from patients with Guillain-Barré syndrome. *Ann Neurol.* 1982;11:69–75.
35. Harrison BM, Hansen LA, Pollard JD, McLeod JG. Demyelination induced by serum from patients with Guillain-Barré syndrome. *Ann Neurol.* 1984;15:163–170.
36. Brown MJ, Rosen JL, Lisak RP. Demyelination in vivo by Guillain-Barré syndrome and other human serum. *Muscle Nerve.* 1987;10:263–271.
37. Sumner AJ. The physiological basis for symptoms in Guillain-Barré syndrome. *Ann Neurol.* 1981;9(suppl):28–30.

38. Liu HM. Ultrastructure of remyelination of peripheral nerves in Landry-Guillain-Barré syndrome. *Acta Neuropathol.* 1970;16:262–265.
39. Vital C, Vallat J-M. Inflammatory polyneuritis. In: *Ultrastructural study of the human diseased peripheral nerve.* New York: Elsevier; 1987:125–147.
40. Wexler I. Sequence of demyelination-remyelination in Guillain-Barré disease. *J Neurol Neurosurg Psychiatry.* 1983;46:168–174.
41. Berger AR, Logigian EL, Shahani BT. Reversible proximal conduction block underlies rapid recovery in Guillain-Barré syndrome. *Muscle Nerve.* 1988;11:1039–1042.
42. Saida K, Sumner AJ, Saida T, Brown MJ, Silberberg DH. Antiserum-mediated demyelination: relationship between remyelination and functional recovery. *Ann Neurol.* 1980;8:12–24.
43. Prineas JW. Demyelination and remyelination in recurrent idiopathic polyneuropathy. An electron microscopic study. *Acta Neuropathol.* 1971;18:34–57.
44. Prineas JW, McLeod JG. Chronic relapsing polyneuritis. *J Neurol Sci.* 1976;27:427–458.
45. Feasby TE, Gilbert JJ, Brown WF, et al. An acute axonal form of Guillain-Barré polyneuropathy. *Brain.* 1986;109:1115–1126.
46. Vallat J-M, Hugon J, Tabaraud F, Leboutet MJ, Chazot F, Dumas M. Quatre cas du syndrome de Guillain-Barré avec lesions axonales. *Rev Neurol.* 1990;146:420–424.
47. Yuki N, Yoshino H, Sato S, Miyatake T. Acute axonal polyneuropathy associated with anti-GM1 antibodies following Campylobacter enteritis. *Neurology.* 1990;40:1900–1902.

9

Immunopathology of Guillain-Barré Syndrome

J.D. Pollard, Ph.D., B.Sc.(Med.), F.R.A.C.P.

The cause of Guillain-Barré syndrome (GBS) is unknown. The pathological changes described in Chapter 8 suggest a delayed hypersensitivity, cell-mediated process. Other features of the disease (e.g., response to plasmapheresis) indicate a role for pathogenic humoral factors. It is likely that the immunopathology of GBS involves complex cellular and humoral pathways that are triggered by some preceding event, most commonly a viral infection. This relationship between GBS and the preceding event is clearly a crucial one, but poorly understood. Most authorities believe that the demyelinating process is an autoimmune disorder triggered by the virus rather than the result of virus invasion of the myelin-producing Schwann cell.[1]

Experimental Allergic Neuritis

The strongest evidence for the belief that GBS represents an autoimmune disorder of peripheral nerve is provided by the close resemblance it shares with experimental allergic neuritis (EAN).[2] This disorder may be induced in animals of many species by homologous or heterologous nerve or nerve antigen. In the species most frequently studied, the Lewis rat, the principal neuritogen is the P_2 basic protein,[3,4] although the more abundant P_0 protein, when changed in conformation by lysophosphatidylcholine, may also produce disease.[5] The activity of P_2 also depends on its conformation; activity is enhanced when P_2 is administered with lipids such as phosphatidyl serine[6] and nuclear magnetic resonance (NMR) studies have shown changes in conformation induced by the lipid. P_2 protein comprises 131 amino acids, but the neuritogenic determinant probably resides in a small polypeptide. Uyemura et al.[7] reported that a synthetic peptide comprising residues 66–78 was neuritogenic but this was not confirmed by Whitaker and Seyser.[8] Shin et al.[9] found the neuritogenic determinant was contained within residues 62–78 but not within 66–78, which indicates that some or all of the residues 62–65 (Ile-Ser-Phe-Lys) are necessary for EAN production. Kadlubowski et al.[10] have studied the localization of P_2 protein in several species and have shown that it is present in highest concentration in the ventral roots, which is the major site of pathological involvement in EAN and GBS.

The clinical course of EAN in the rat is usually monophasic, as is GBS, but relapses may be seen after a single immunization depending on the dose of neuritogen and the period of follow-up.[11,12] In the rabbit a chronic relapsing form of disease is easily produced by a single inoculation with a large dose of antigen.[13] This spectrum of clinical manifestations of EAN lends support to the view that GBS and its chronic variant, chronic inflammatory demyelinating polyradiculoneuropathy (CIDP), are part of a single disease process.

Cellular Immunity in EAN

The pathology of EAN, like that of GBS, is highly suggestive of a delayed hypersensitivity, cell-mediated response (DTH); myelin is removed by macrophage-monocytes, the dominant inflammatory cell within the endoneurium[14] (Fig. 9–1), although T cells, both W3/25 (helper) and OX8 (suppressor), are present.[15] The role of cellular immunity in EAN has been strongly supported by experimental studies involving passive transfer. Arnason and Chelmicka-Szorc[16] produced demyelinating lesions within nerve by intraneural injection of EAN lymph node cells into isogeneic animals. More recently, adoptive transfer of disease has been achieved using T-cell lines reactive to P_2.[17,18] Brosnan et al.[19] have, moreover, shown that T cell–deficient rats (following thymectomy and irradiation) are less susceptible to disease induction. However, it is not yet understood how these T cells enter nerve and cause demyelination. Lymphocytes have been shown to accumulate within venules and then traverse these shortly before clinical signs of disease, and before the accumulation of macrophages within the nerve.[20] Presumably the latter cell is recruited by lymphokines and other factors released by lymphocytes. Several recent studies have emphasized the important role of macrophages in the demyelinating process. Experiments using silica dust to inactivate macrophages showed suppression of EAN.[21-23] Since macrophages can form highly reactive oxygen metabolites, such as superoxide anion and

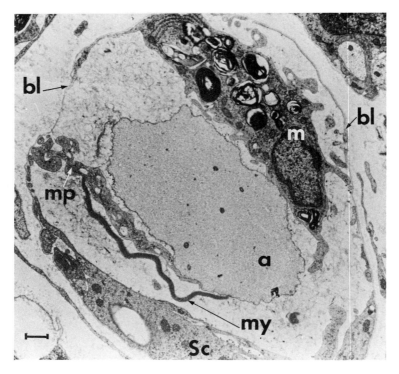

Figure 9–1.   An electron micrograph illustrating the demyelinating process in EAN. A macrophage (*M*) containing myelin debris has entered the Schwann cell basal lamina (*bl*) and engulfed the myelin sheath, leaving a large naked axon (*a*). A macrophage process (*mp*) is seen removing the final remnant of the myelin sheath (*my*). *Sc*, Schwann cell cytoplasm; Bar = 1 μm.

hydrogen peroxide, Hartung et al.[23] treated EAN rats with oxygen radical scavengers, superoxide dismutase, and catelase and observed marked suppression of disease activity, a result that implies involvement of macrophage-derived oxidants in the demyelinating process of EAN. The same workers[24] examined the role of other macrophage products and have assessed inhibition of eicosanoid mediators in EAN. They found inhibition of the cyclooxygenase pathway with Indomethacin or BW755c (Wellcome) suppressed EAN whereas no suppression was achieved by inhibition of the lipoxygenase pathway. Macrophages are also a potent source of proteases, minute quantities of which, when injected intraneurally, have been shown to produce widespread demyelination[25,26] (Fig. 9–2).

Antigen Presentation

Before a DTH response can occur in peripheral nerve, the antigen (P₂) must be presented to CD4 (W3/25) lymphocytes within nerve. Cells capable of pre-

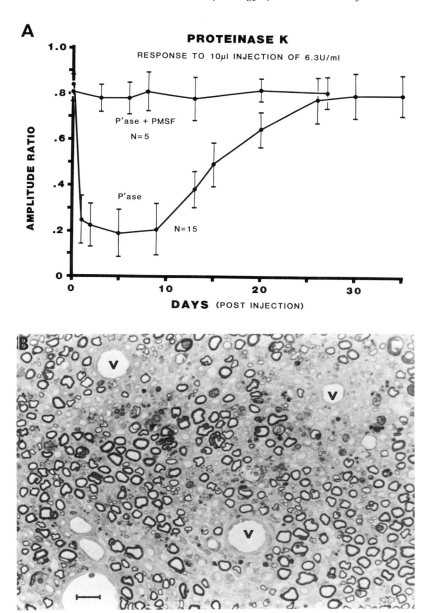

Figure 9–2. The effect of intraneural protease injection in rat tibial nerve. **A**: Electrophysiological changes. Proteinase alone produces rapid and profound conduction block, shown by marked fall in the ratio of compound muscle action potential amplitudes following stimulation proximal and distal to injection site (amplitude ratio). Proteinase combined with specific inhibitor PMSF has no effect. Note the similarity to Fig. 9–5. **B**: Histological changes. A transverse section of injected nerve stained with toluidine blue to show myelinated fibers. Note marked perivascular demyelination. *V*, blood vessels (endoneurial capillaries); Bar = 10 μm.

senting and processing antigen, antigen-presenting cells (APC), usually express constitutively high levels of Class II major histocompatibility (MHC) molecules on their surface. In many tissues, such cells have been shown to be resident dendritic cells, or macrophages. However, recent studies have shown that Schwann cells (Scs), although they normally do not express Class II MHC, can be induced to do so by lymphokines such as interferon-gamma (IFN-G)[27–29] (Fig. 9–3). Wekerle et al.[27] have shown *in vitro* that Scs can present neural antigen and interact with syngeneic autoaggressive T cells. These functions were blocked by anti-Ia antibody. Armati et al.[29] have shown Class II MHC not only on the surface of Scs incubated with IFN-G but also within endosomes within the cells, a finding consistent with current concepts of antigen-presenting and -processing cells. Immunocytochemical studies have shown not only W3/25 and OX8 positive T cells within EAN nerve,[15] but also ED1 positive macrophages[24] and increased expression of Class I and II MHC.[15,30] Schafer et al.[31] have treated EAN rats with recombinant IFN-G and found that when given in the induction phase of disease (days 1–10), marked enhancement of disease expression was seen. Whether this effect results from increased MHC expression on Scs and other cells, from heightened macrophage activation, increased permeability of vascular endothelium, or other immunomodulatory effects of IFN-G is not yet known. In recent *in vitro* studies Tsai et al.[32] have shown that syngeneic P_2-responsive T cells are at least as effective as IFN-G in inducing Class I and II MHC molecules on Scs and that these T cells cluster around the Scs in a manner characteristic of antigen presentation[33,34] (Fig. 9–4). Moreover, the use of inhibitors of IFN-G including dibutyryl cyclic adenosine monophosphate (cAMP), prostaglandin E_2, methylxanthine, cyclosporine A, or hydrocortisone can effectively prevent the Sc expression of MHC whether induced by recombinant IFN-G or reactive T cells, and under such circumstances the T cells no longer cluster around the T cells.[32] Disease suppression in EAN animals was achieved by treatment with dibutyryl cAMP and a phosphodiesterase inhibitor (aminophylline) to inhibit IFN-G.

Humoral Mechanisms in EAN

Considerable interest in this area followed the finding of Saida et al.[35] that the intraneural injection of rabbit EAN serum produced profound demyelination in rat sciatic nerve (Fig. 9–5). Most of this demyelinating activity is due to antibodies to galactocerebroside[36–38] (Fig. 9–6). EAN may also be induced in rabbits after inoculation with galactocerebroside (GC) and all affected rabbits have elevated levels of anti-GC antibody.[37] GC-induced neuropathy is regarded as an antibody-mediated disease and occurs mainly at sites of blood–nerve barrier deficiency. Antibody to P_2, however, does not produce demyelination when injected into rat nerve even though anti-P_2 antibody is found in rats with EAN. In addition to anti-GC antibody, antibody to P_0 also causes demyelination[39] when injected intraneurally.

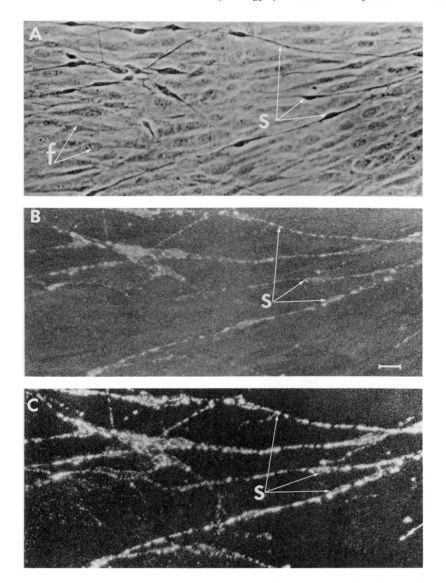

Figure 9–3. Class II MHC expression on rat Schwann cells *in vitro*, treated with recombinant interferon gamma 100 IU/ml. **A**: Phase contrast of rat dorsal root ganglia cultures 7 DIV; *S,* Schwann cell; *F,* fibroblast. **B**: The same culture immunostained with 217C (fluorescein-labeled) to identify Schwann cells (*S*). **C**: Immunostained with monoclonal antibody to rat class II (OX6) (Texas red labeled). Note only Schwann cells (217C positive cells) are positive for MHC class II. Bar = 20 μm.

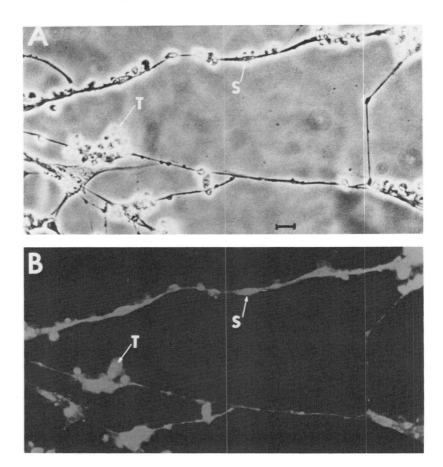

Figure 9–4.   Clustering of P_2-responsive T cells to Schwann cells *in vitro*. **A**: Phase contrast of rat dorsal root ganglia cultures cocultured with P_2-responsive T cells. Note T cells (*T*) are all clustered along Schwann cells (*S*). **B**: As above, immunostained with monoclonal antibody to rat MHC class II (OX6) (Texas red labeled). Bar = 20 μm.

Further evidence for humoral mechanisms is provided by the finding of Feasby et al.[40] that complement depletion by cobra venom treatment suppresses EAN.

Humoral Mechanisms in GBS

Evidence for Antibody

Despite strong evidence of pathogenic antibody to defined antigens in EAN, there is no such evidence that antibodies to P_2, P_0, or GC play a role in the

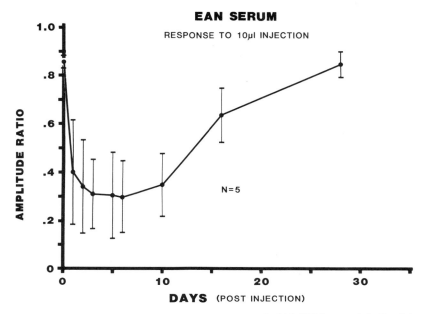

Figure 9–5. Electrophysiological changes after intraneural rabbit EAN serum injection into rat tibial nerve. Injection of EAN serum produces rapid and profound conduction block shown by a fall in the ratio of compound muscle action potential amplitudes after stimulation proximal and distal to injection site.

human disease.[41,42] Cook and Dowling[43] reviewed the early evidence for autoantibody in GBS; they summarized a considerable number of reports in which several different assay systems were used, but in many studies there was a lack of specificity since antibody was also found in some normal patients.

Interest in antibody mechanisms was increased when Feasby et al.[44] and Sumner et al.[45] demonstrated that GBS serum demyelinated rat sciatic nerve and could produce rapid conduction block, when injected intraneurally. Although other workers disputed this effect,[46] the differences may be attributed to different methods of storage, since Harrison et al.[47] found demyelinating activity was lost on prolonged storage. Attempts to produce demyelination by passive transfer of human serum to immunosuppressed mice or primates have, however, been largely unsuccessful.[48]

Nyland and Aarli[49] found specific IgG binding to peripheral nerve, in 15 of 30 cases of GBS, in a study employing the antibody consumption test. All controls were negative. Since 1985 Koski and her coworkers[50] have consistently demonstrated complement-fixing antibodies to peripheral nerve myelin in the serum of GBS patients. These antibodies correlate with disease activity; they are highest when neurologic symptoms first occur and are

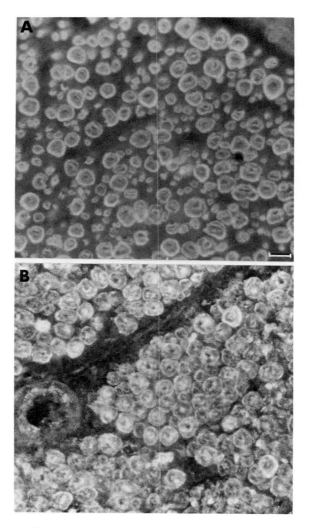

Figure 9–6. Immunofluorescent studies of nerve, showing antibody binding to myelin sheaths. **A**: A transverse section of rat sciatic nerve incubated in rabbit EAN serum and then immunostained to show antimyelin immunoglobulin. **B**: Normal human sural nerve incubated in serum from a plasma exchange responsive GBS patient and then immunostained to show anti-C3 antibody. Bar = 10 μm.

cleared as the clinical status improves.[51] Moreover, they correlate with the appearance of activated products of the terminal complement cascade in serum, cerebrospinal fluid, and peripheral nerve of GBS patients.[52–54] (Fig. 9–6).

In a post mortem study of a GBS patient, evidence was found of C_3, C_9, and IgM on nerve root and peripheral nerve.[54] It would appear that anti-peripheral nerve myelin (PNM) antibodies in GBS serum bind to human PNM and activate complement, thus generating C_3, C_{5a}, and C_{5b-9}, which may contribute to demyelination. Recent studies suggest that the target antigen within PNM for these antibodies is a myelin lipid; Ilyas et al.[55] found 6 of 21 GBS sera contained IgM and/or IgG antibodies that bound to carbohydrate determinants in a series of peripheral and central nerve myelin gangliosides. Koski et al.[56] found all GBS sera tested reacted with a neutral glycolipid of PNM that cross-reacted with Forssman hapten.

Other Circulating Factors

The response to plasma exchange of patients with GBS or CIDP provides cogent evidence for the operation of humoral mechanisms in these disorders, but clearly many factors apart from antibody may be removed by this therapy. The process of inflammation is exceedingly complex; lymphocytes produce soluble factors, lymphokines, that can modulate the inflammatory response at many levels. Macrophages likewise produce toxic products, oxygen free radicals, proteases, and eicosanoids, and serum abounds in other proinflammatory mediators including complement components. These and other factors may regulate cell-mediated responses, so that response to plasma exchange does not of itself illuminate the pathogenesis of inflammatory demyelinating neuropathy.

Cell-Mediated Mechanisms in GBS

Although the pathology of GBS, like that of EAN, is strongly suggestive of a cell-mediated hypersensitivity response, T-cell hyperresponsiveness to P_2, GC, or any other defined neural antigen has not been consistently demonstrated.[41,42,57] Several earlier reports described T-cell activation to crude peripheral nerve fractions, using different assays including macrophage migration inhibition, leukocyte inhibitory factor assay, and tritiated thymidine uptake,[58–60] but these findings have not been confirmed when purified neuritogens have been used.[41]

In studies of circulating T-cell subsets in GBS, conflicting results have been obtained; Hauser et al.[61] found no significant change in the CD4/CD8 cell ratio; Hughes et al.[62] and Lisak et al.[63] reported abnormalities in this ratio. Such ratios are probably of more significance in the target organ, but few studies have been reported. Cornblath et al.[64] found the CD4/CD8 ratio in nerve reflected that of the peripheral blood in four cases studied.

Pollard et al.[65] found no significant difference in the CD4/CD8 ratio in two cases but confirmed earlier electron microscope studies that showed that the dominant infiltrating cell was the macrophage/monocyte.[66] Moreover, there is a marked increase in MHC Class I and II in GBS nerve in regions showing demyelination and this increase is in excess of that resulting from the mononuclear cell infiltrate (Fig. 9–7). Immunoelectron microscopy localized the MHC molecules to the surface of endothelial cells, invading mononuclear cells and Schwann cells (Fig. 9–8). These findings then are in keeping with *in vitro* studies,[28,29] which have shown MHC Class I and II on human Schwann cells after incubation with IFN-G or reactive T cells, and raise the possibility that the Schwann cell may play an active role in inflammatory demyelinating neuropathy as a target for T-cell attack or as an antigen-presenting cell.

Immunogenetic Studies

No definite association has been shown between GBS and antigens of the HLA system.[67,68] A possible association with HLA DR2 has, however, been recently reported for cases of CIDP.[69] McCombe et al.[70] found an association for both GBS and CIDP with the M3 allele of alpha-1-antitrypsin, the major serum proteinase inhibitor.

Because of the linkage that is known to occur on chromosome 14 between alpha-1-antitrypsin and genes that code for constant regions of IgG heavy chains (GM), Feeney et al.[71] examined the possible association of GM haplotypes with inflammatory demyelinating neuropathies and found that GM 1,2,17;21 is significantly overrepresented in patients with GBS and to a lesser extent those with CIDP. Hence in GBS there is at this time evidence for genetic factors affecting immunoglobulin synthesis and proteinase inhibition, two pathways that may well be implicated in the demyelinating process.

Other Animal Models of GBS

Marek's Disease

Marek's disease is an endemic disease of fowl due to an oncogenic Group B herpes virus.[72,73] The fowl develop progressive weakness and paralysis, usually in association with lymphomatous deposits in nerve, uveal tract, brain, abdominal organs, muscle, and skin. Early changes in nerve consist of perivenous demyelination in association with infiltrates of lymphocytes, monocytes, and macrophages, changes very similar to those found in EAN and experimental allergic encephalomyelitis (EAE).[74] Sections through swollen nerve segments show massive infiltrates of mononuclear cells with widespread destruction of myelin and axons and, distal to these areas, active wallerian degeneration is seen. The mechanism of demyelination is similar in all respects to that seen in EAN or GBS, stripping of apparently normal myelin by macrophage processes. The virus can be readily demonstrated in the epithelial cells of the feather follicle, but only with extreme difficulty in other tissues.[75] However, virus can be recovered from lymphoid tumors, nerve, and peripheral blood cells by cocultivation techniques *in vitro*.[73] It is

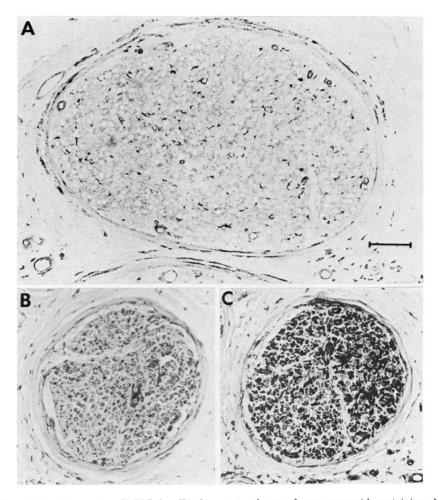

Figure 9–7. Expression of MHC class II in human sural nerve. Immunoperoxidase staining. **A**: Transverse section of sural nerve from a normal patient immunostained to show MHC class II (anti-Ia Coulter). Note reaction product around blood vessels but scantily within endoneurium. **B**: Transverse section. Sural nerve from a GBS patient immunostained to show macrophage-monocytes (FMC-32 Australian Monoclonal Developments). **C**: Adjacent section to B immunostained to show MHC class II (anti-Ia Coulter). Note dense expression of class II far beyond that accounted for by cellular infiltration. Bar = 10 μm.

uncertain whether demyelination in Marek's disease results from direct viral invasion and damage to Schwann cells or by autoimmune mechanisms. The latter appears far more likely since no cytopathic Schwann cell changes have been described and virus particles are not evident in Schwann cells or invading mononuclear cells. The immune response may be directed against

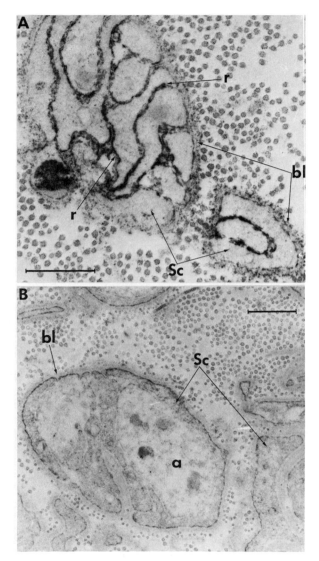

Figure 9–8. Electron micrograph showing MHC class II expression on Schwann cells. **A:** Section of sural nerve from GBS patient immunostained to show MHC class II (anti-Ia Coulter). Immunoperoxidase staining. **B:** Section of sural nerve from a normal control patient immunostained as above. *S.C.*, Schwann cell; *bl*, Schwann cell basal lamina; *A*, axon; *R*, reaction product; Bar = 1 μm.

virus-associated cell surface antigens or against a component of Schwann cell or myelin membrane, through molecular mimickry or a similar mechanism.

Since herpes viruses are commonly involved in antecedent infections to GBS, a better understanding of the relationship of the Marek virus to this demyelinating disease in fowl may well help elucidate demyelinating mechanisms in GBS.

Experimental Chagas' Disease

Said and coworkers[76] have shown that mice chronically infected with *Trypanosoma cruzi* (the causative agent of Chagas' disease) develop multifocal perivascular, granulomatous lesions of nerve that are associated with predominantly demyelinative changes in adjacent nerve fibers. These demyelinating lesions were reproduced by intraneural injections of small numbers of live parasites and by passive transfer of 10^7 helper T cells from infected mice, but not by intraneural injection of serum from such animals. These findings suggest that the nerve lesions result from mechanisms involving delayed hypersensitivity with macrophage-mediated demyelination.

Coonhound Paralysis

Cummings and Haas[77] have described an acute idiopathic polyradiculoneuritis in dogs that occurs 7 to 14 days after a raccoon bite. The clinical disorder is similar to the human disease and repeated episodes may occur after further bites. Although some dogs recover completely, in others severe muscle atrophy, consequent upon axonal degeneration, results. Pathological changes are found throughout the peripheral nervous system but they are maximal in the ventral roots in the lumbosacral region. Segmental demyelination is the basic lesion but axonal damage occurs in some animals. These changes occur in the presence of inflammatory infiltrates, lymphocytes, mononuclear cells, plasma cells, and some polymorphonuclear cells. No virus has been isolated from affected dogs or raccoon saliva.

This condition is clearly similar to GBS in clinical and pathological features and in the period between the illness and initiating event. The failure to show viral infection and the repeated episodes in a single animal suggest that coonhound paralysis is also an autoallergic disorder.

Summary

Although the pathogenesis of GBS remains uncertain, there are several striking and consistent findings that appear to be key issues. The first of these is the frequent precipitation by viral infections. Certain patients with the related chronic relapsing demyelinating neuropathy regularly and predictably suffer repeated attacks after viral infection. It is highly unlikely that the many viruses or other events that have been associated with GBS would all invade peripheral nerve and damage the Schwann cell. It would seem more likely that some molecular mimickry is involved between the infectious agent and a Schwann cell/myelin antigen and/or the virus, or other agent, produces a nonspecific arousal of immune responses. Viral infections are known to induce interferon production by T cells. IFN-G may induce MHC Class I and II on many cell types including vascular endothelium[78] and Schwann cells; it may increase permeability of endothelium to T cells and macrophages and increase activation of macrophages. Circulating reactive T cells (CD4) may thus traverse the blood–nerve barrier and recognize neural antigen in association with Class II MHC on Schwann cells. T-cell proliferation may then result in a DTH reaction with recruitment of activated macrophages that result in myelin destruction. Alternatively, cytotoxic CD8 T cells may target and damage MHC Class I positive Schwann cells that can no longer maintain myelin, which is then removed by macrophages.

That the macrophage appears to be the main effector cell in GBS is the second constant finding in this disease. In addition, through a similar initial process of cross immunization, antibody produced to infectious agents could bind to peripheral nerve myelin and participate in the demyelinating process. Such a synergistic response has recently been demonstrated in experimental allergic encephalomyelitis, when this T cell–mediated disease shows enhanced demyelination by the systemic administration of antibody to oligodendrocyte-associated glycoprotein.

The third striking feature of GBS is the overwhelming evidence for the efficacy of plasmapheresis. Unfortunately, this does not enlighten the uncertain pathogenesis of this disease since the benefits of plasmapheresis could result from effects at many levels: removal of antibody, lymphokine, or toxic cell product or by all of these.

References

1. Arnason BWG. Acute inflammatory demyelinating polyradiculoneuropathy. In: Dyck PJ, Thomas PK, Lampert PW, Bunge R, eds. *Peripheral Neuropathy*. London: Saunders; 1984: 2050–2100.
2. Waksman BH, Adams RD. Allergic neuritis: experimental disease of rabbits induced by the injection of peripheral nervous tissue and adjuvants. *J Exp Med*. 1955;102:213–235.
3. Brostoff SW, Levitt S, Powers JM. Induction of experimental allergic neuritis with a peptide from myelin P_2 basic protein. *Nature (Lond.)*. 1977;268:752–753.
4. Kadlubowski M, Hughes RAC. Identification of the neuritogen for experimental allergic neuritis. *Nature*. 1979;277:140–141.
5. Milner PCA, Loverlidge WA, Taylor WA, Hughes RAC. P_2 protein in peripheral nerve myelin. *J Neurochem*. 1987;39:895–898.
6. Curtis BM, Forno LS, Smith ME. Reactivation of neuritogenic activity of P_2 protein from rabbit PNS myelin. *Brain Res*. 1979;175:387–391.
7. Uyemura K, Suzuki M, Kitamura K, et al. Neuritogenic determinant of bovine P_2 protein in peripheral nerve myelin. *J Neurochem*. 1982;39:895–898.
8. Whitaker J, Seyser J. Degradation of bovine P_2 protein by bovine brain cathepsin D. *Neurochem Res*. 1984;9:1431–1443.

9. Shin H-C, McFarlane EF, Pollard JD, Watson EGS. Induction of experimental allergic neuritis with synthetic peptides from myelin P_2 protein. *Neurosci Lett.* 1989;102:309–312.
10. Kadlubowski M, Hughes RAC, Gregson NA. Spontaneous and experimental neuritis and the distribution of the myelin protein P_2 in the nervous system. *J Neurochem.* 1984;42: 123–129.
11. Brosnan CF, Lyman WD, Neighbour PA. Chronic experimental allergic neuritis in the Lewis rat. *J Neuropathol Exp Neurol.* 1984;43:302. Abstract.
12. Craggs RI, Brosnan JV, King RHM, Thomas PK. Chronic relapsing experimental allergic neuritis in Lewis rats. Effects of thymectomy and splenectomy. *Acta Neuropathol.* 1986;70: 22–29.
13. Harvey GK, Pollard JD, Schindhelm K, Antony J. Chronic experimental allergic neuritis. An electrophysiological and histological study in the rabbit. *J Neurol Sci.* 1987;81:215–225.
14. Lampert PW. Mechanisms of demyelination in experimental allergic neuritis—electromicroscopic studies. *Lab Invest.* 1969;20:127–138.
15. Olsson T, Holmdahl R, Klareskog L, Forsum U, Kristensson K. Dynamics of Ia-expressing cells and T lymphocytes of different subsets during experimental allergic neuritis in Lewis rats. *J Neurol Sci.* 1984;66:141–149.
16. Arnason BGW, Chelmicka-Szorc E. Passive transfer of experimental allergic neuritis in Lewis rats by direct injection of sensitized lymphocytes into sciatic nerves. *Acta Neuropathol.* 1972;22:1–6.
17. Linington C, Izumo S, Suzuki M, Uyemura K, Wekerle H. A permanent rat T cell line that mediates experimental allergic neuritis in the Lewis rat in vivo. *J Immunol.* 1984;133:1946–1950.
18. Rostami A, Burns JB, Brown MJ, et al. Transfer of experimental allergic neuritis with P_2-reactive T-cell lines. *Cell Immunol.* 1985;91:354–361.
19. Brosnan JV, Craggs RI, King RH, Thomas PK. Reduced susceptibility of T cell-deficient rats to induction of experimental allergic neuritis. *J Neuroimmunol.* 1987;14:267–282.
20. Astrom KE, Webster H de F, Arnason BGW. The initial lesion in experimental allergic neuritis. *J Exp Med.* 1968;128:469–481.
21. Tansey FA, Brosnan CF. Protection against experimental allergic neuritis with silica quartz dust. *J Neuroimmunol.* 1983;3:169–179.
22. Craggs RL, King RHM, Thomas PK. The effect of suppression of macrophage activity on the development of experimental allergic neuritis. *Acta Neuropathol.* 1984;62:316–232.
23. Hartung HP, Schafer B, Heininger K, Toyka KV. Suppression of experimental autoimmune neuritis by the oxygen radical scavengers, superoxide dismutase and catalase. *Ann Neurol.* 1988;23:453–460.
24. Hartung HP, Schafer B, Heininger K, Stoll G, Toyka KV. The role of macrophages and eicosanoids in the pathogenesis of experimental allergic neuritis. Serial clinical, electrophysiological, biochemical, and morphological observations. *Brain.* 1988;111:1039–1059.
25. Gross JL, Jenson J, Said G, Sumner AJ. An experimental model of proteinase induced focal demyelination. *Neurology.* 1984;34:131. Abstract.
26. Westland K, Pollard JD. Proteinase induced demyelination. An electrophysiological and histological study. *J Neurol Sci.* 1987;82:41–53.
27. Wekerle H, Schwab M, Linington C, Meyermann R. Antigen presentation in the peripheral nervous system: Schwann cells present endogenous myelin autoantigens to lymphocytes. *Eur J Immunol.* 1986;16:1551–1557.
28. Samuel NM, Jessen KR, Grange JM, Mirsky R. Gamma interferon, but not Mycobacterium leprae, induces major histocompatibility Class II antigens on cultured rat Schwann cells. *J Neurocytol.* 1987;16:282–287.
29. Armati PJ, Pollard JD, Gatenby P. Rat and human Schwann cells in vitro can synthesize and express MHC Class I and II molecules. *Muscle Nerve.* 1990;113:110–116.
30. Hughes RAC, Atkinson PF, Gray IA, Taylor WA. Major histo-compatibility antigens and lymphocyte subsets during experimental allergic neuritis in the Lewis rat. *J Neurol.* 1987; 234:390–395.
31. Schafer B, Hartung HP, Heininger K, Van der Meide PH, Blomenkamp G, Toyka KV. Modulation of experimental autoimmune neuritis by recombinant interferon gamma. *J Neurol.* 1988;235(suppl.):S64.
32. Tsai CP, Pollard JD, Armati PJ. Interferon-gamma inhibition suppresses EAN: modulation of major HC complex expression of Schwann cells in vitro. *J Neuroimmunol.* 1991;31:133–145.
33. Fontana A, Erb P, Pircher H, Zinkernagel R, Weber E, Fierz W. Astrocytes as antigen-

presenting cells. Part II: Unlike H-2K-Dependent Cytotoxic T cells, H-21a-Restricted T cells are only stimulated in the presence of interferon-y. *J Neuroimmunol*. 1986;12:15–28.

34. Kingston AE, Bergsteinsdottir K, Jessen KR, Van der Meide PH, Colston JM, Mirsky R. Schwann cells co-cultured with stimulated T cells and antigen express major histocompatibility complex (MHC) Class II determinants without interferon gamma pretreatment: synergistic effects of interferon gamma and tumour necrosis factor on MHC Class II induction. *Eur J Immunol*. 1989;19:177–183.

35. Saida T, Saida K, Silberberg DH, Brown MJ. Transfer of demyelination with experimental allergic neuritis serum by intraneural injection. *Nature*. 1978;272:639–641.

36. Saida K, Saida T, Brown MJ, Silberberg DJ. In vivo demyelination induced by intraneural injection of anti-galactocerebroside serum. *Am J Pathol*. 1979;95:99–116.

37. Saida T, Saida K, Dorfman S, et al. Experimental allergic neuritis induced by sensitization with galactocerebroside. *Science*. 1979;204:1103–1106.

38. Saida T, Saida K, Silberberg DH, Brown MJ. Experimental allergic neuritis induced by galactocerebroside. *Ann Neurol*. 1981;9(suppl):87–91.

39. Hughes RAC, Powell HC, Braheny SL, Brostoff S. Endoneurial injection of antisera to myelin antigens. *Muscle Nerve*. 1985;8:516–522.

40. Feasby TE, Gilbert JJ, Hahn AF, Neilson M. Complement depletion suppresses Lewis rat experimental allergic neuritis. *Brain Res*. 1987;419:97–103.

41. Hughes RAC, Gray IA, Gregson NA, et al. Immune responses to myelin antigens in Guillain-Barré syndrome. *J Neuroimmunol*. 1984;6:303–312.

42. Zweiman B, Rostami A, Lisak RP, Moskovitz AR, Pleasure DE. Immune reactions to P_2 protein in human inflammatory demyelinative neuropathies. *Neurology*. 1983;33:234–237.

43. Cook SD, Dowling PC. The role of autoantibody and immune complexes in the pathogenesis of Guillain-Barré syndrome. *Ann Neurol*. 1981;9(suppl):70–79.

44. Feasby TE, Hahn AF, Gilbert JJ. Passive transfer studies in Guillain-Barré polyneuropathy. *Neurology*. 1982;32:1159–1167.

45. Sumner AJ, Saïd G, Idy I, Metral S. Syndrome de Guillain-Barré: effets electrophysiologiques et morphologiques du serum humain introduit dans l'espace endoneural du nerf sciatique du rat: resultats preliminaires. *Rev Neurol (Paris)*. 1982;138:17–24.

46. Low PA, Schmelzer J, Dyck PJ, Kelly JJ. Endoneurial effects of sera from patients with acute inflammatory polyradiculoneuropathy: electrophysiologic studies on normal and demyelinated rat nerves. *Neurology*. 1982;32:720–724.

47. Harrison BM, Hansen LA, Pollard JD, McLeod JG. Demyelination induced by serum from patients with Guillain-Barré syndrome. *Ann Neurol*. 1989;15:163–170.

48. Toyka KV, Heininger K. Humoral factors in peripheral nerve disease. *Muscle Nerve*. 1987;10:222–232.

49. Nyland J, Aarli JA. Guillain-Barré syndrome: demonstration of antibodies to peripheral nerve tissue. *Acta Neurol Scand*. 1978;58:35–43.

50. Koski CL, Humphrey R, Shin MS. Anti-peripheral myelin antibody in patients with demyelinating neuropathy: quantitative and kinetic determination of serum antibody by complement component 1 fixation. *Proc Natl Acad Sci USA*. 1985;82:905–909.

51. Koski CL, Gratz E, Sutherland J, Mayer RF. Clinical correlation with anti-peripheral-nerve myelin antibodies in Guillain-Barré syndrome. *Ann Neurol*. 1986;19:573–577.

52. Sanders ME, Koski CL, Robbins D, Shin ML, Frank MM, Joinrt KA. Activated terminal complement in cerebrospinal fluid in Guillain-Barré syndrome and multiple sclerosis. *J Immunol*. 1986;136:4456–4459.

53. Hartung HP, Schwenke C, Bitter Swermann D, Toyka KV. Activated terminal complement C_{36} and C_{5-9} in cerebrospinal fluid in terminal complement in Guillain-Barré syndrome. *Neurology*. 1986;37:1006–1009.

54. Koski CL, Sandes ME, Swoveland PT, et al. Activation of terminal components of complement in patients with Guillain-Barré syndrome and other demyelinating neuropathies. *J Clin Invest*. 1987;80:1492–1497.

55. Ilyas AA, Willison HJ, Quarles RH, et al. Serum antibodies to gangliosides in Guillain-Barré syndrome. *Ann Neurol*. 1988;23:440–447.

56. Koski CL, Chou DKH, Jungalwala FB. Anti-peripheral nerve myelin antibodies in Guillain-Barré syndrome bind a neutral glycolipid of peripheral myelin and cross-react with Forssman antigen. *J Clin Invest*. 1989;84:280–287.

57. Iqbal A, Oger JJ-F, Arnason BGW. Cell-mediated immunity in idiopathic polyneuritis. *Ann Neurol*. 1981;9(suppl):65–69.

58. Behan PO, Lamarche JB, Feldman RG, Sheremata WA. Lymphocyte transformation in the Guillain-Barré syndrome. *Lancet.* 1970;1:421.
59. Castaigne P, Berthaux P, Brunet P, Moulias R, Goust J-M, Delrieu F. Polyradiculonevrites inflammatoires et immunite cellulaire: etude de la reponse immunitaire cellulaire envers des antigens de nerf peripherique par le test de migration des leucocytes. *Nouv Presse Med.* 1972; 1:2445–2449.
60. Sheremata W, Colby S, Lusky G, Cosgrove JBR. Cellular hypersensitization to peripheral nervous antigens in the Guillain-Barré syndrome. *Neurology.* 1975;25:833–839.
61. Hauser SL, Ropper AH, Perlo VP, Reinherz EL, Schlossmann SF, Weiner HS. T-cell subsets in human autoimmune diseases. *Neurology.* 1982;32:1321–1322.
62. Hughes RAC, Aslan S, Gray IA. Lymphocyte subpopulations and suppressor cell activity in acute polyradiculoneuritis (Guillain-Barré syndrome). *Clin Exp Immunol.* 1983;51:448–454.
63. Lisak RP, Zweiman B, Guerrero F, Moskovitz AR. Circulating T-cell subsets in Guillain-Barré syndrome. *J Neuroimmunol.* 1985;8:93–101.
64. Cornblath DR, Griffin DE, Chupp M, Griffin JW, McArthur JC. Mononuclear cell typing in inflammatory demyelinating polyneuropathy nerve biopsies. *Neurology.* 1987;37:253. Abstract.
65. Pollard JD, Baverstock J, McLeod JG. Class II antigen expression and inflammatory cells in the Guillain-Barré syndrome. *Ann Neurol.* 1987;21:337–341.
66. Prineas JW. Acute idiopathic polyneuritis. An electron microscope study. *Lab Invest.* 1972; 26:133–141.
67. Adams D, Gibson JD, Thomas PK, et al. HLA antigens in Guillain-Barré syndrome. *Lancet.* 1977;2:504–505.
68. Stewart GJ, Pollard JD, McLeod JG, Wolinzer CM. HLA antigens in the Landry-Guillain-Barré syndrome and chronic relapsing polyneuritis. *Ann Neurol.* 1978;4:285–289.
69. Feeney DJ, Pollard JD, McLeod JG, Stewart GJ, Doran TJ. HLA antigens in chronic inflammatory demyelinating polyneuropathy. *J Neurol Neurosurg Psychiatry.* 1990;53:170–172.
70. McCombe PA, Clark P, Frith JA, et al. α-1 antitrypsin phenotypes in demyelinating disease: an association between demyelinating disease and the allele PiM3. *Ann Neurol.* 1985;18: 514–516.
71. Feeney DJ, Pollard JD, McLeod JG, Stewart GJ, Delange GG. GM haplotyes in inflammatory demyelinating neuropathies. *Ann Neurol.* 1989;26:790–792.
72. Marek J. Multiple nervenetzundung (polyneuritis) bei huhnern. *Dtsch Tieraztl Wochenschr.* 1907;15:417–421.
73. Churchill AE, Briggs PM. Agent of Marek's disease in tissue culture. *Nature (Lond.).* 1967;245:528.
74. Prineas JW, Wright RG. The time structure of peripheral nerve lesions in a virus induced demyelinating disease of fowl (Marek's disease). *Lab Invest.* 1972;26:548–557.
75. Calrek BW, Ubertine T, Adlinger HK. Viral antigen, virus particles and infectivity of tissues from chickens with Marek's disease. *J Natl Cancer Inst.* 1970;45:341–347.
76. Said G, Joskowicz M, Barreira AA, Eisen H. Neuropathy associated with experimental Chagas disease. *Ann Neurol.* 1985;18:676–683.
77. Cummings JF, Haas DC. Coonhound paralysis. An acute idiopathic polyradiculoneuritis in dogs resembling the Landry-Guillain-Barré syndrome. *J Neurol Sci.* 1967;4:51–81.
78. Pober JS, Collins T, Gimbrone MA, et al. Lymphocytes recognize human vascular endothelium and dermal fibroblast in antigens induced by recombinant immune interferon. *Nature.* 1983;305:726–729.
79. Linington C, Bradl M, Lassmann H, Brunner C, Vass K. Augmentation of demyelination in rat acute allergic encephalomyelitis by circulating mouse monoclonal antibodies against a myelin-oligodendrocyte glycoprotein. *Am J Pathol.* 1988;130:443–454.

10

Chronic Inflammatory Demyelinating Polyradiculoneuropathy

Chronic inflammatory demyelinating polyradiculoneuropathy (CIDP) is an idiopathic, acquired demyelinating neuropathy that shares many clinical, electrophysiological, and pathological features with Guillain-Barré syndrome (GBS). It differs chiefly by virtue of its rate of evolution, its prognosis, and to some extent, by its response to treatment. Indeed, 15% to 20% of cases of CIDP have an acute presentation virtually indistinguishable from GBS and the initial attack may even resolve spontaneously and completely, only to relapse at a later date. Conversely, some degree of relapse during the recovery phase of GBS, although uncommon, does occur in about 5% of patients with otherwise typical disease and does not appear to predict progression to CIDP. The factors that determine the differences in the course of these two closely related autoimmune neuropathies are largely obscure.

The entire range of the subject of CIDP and the other chronic acquired demyelinating neuropathies is a large one and is beyond the scope of this chapter; I will highlight those areas in which CIDP resembles GBS and will compare and contrast these two closely related disorders. I will describe the features in 30 patients seen at the Louisiana State University (LSU) Medical

Center in New Orleans and compare them with those described in three large series totalling more than 200 cases reported in the literature.[1–3] Since the disease appears to behave differently in children, I have separated adults from children (<16 years of age). CIDP has been defined as an acquired neuropathy in which there is unequivocal evidence of demyelination as the primary pathology. The presence of demyelination has been established electrophysiologically, using the criteria elaborated by the American Academy of Neurology, AIDS Task Force,[4] and in some cases pathologically. Patients in whom another cause of neuropathy has been identified, such as diabetes, renal failure, exposure to neurotoxins, and all patients with familial neuropathy have been excluded. Also excluded are all patients with serum paraproteinemia, including those with IgM paraproteinemia with antibodies to myelin-associated glycoprotein. Finally, I have excluded patients with multifocal motor neuropathy, despite its many similarities with CIDP, since this disorder may represent a distinct nosological entity.

Clinical Features

Course and Evolution

The major difference between GBS and CIDP is the temporal profile of these diseases. In most of the CIDP patients at LSU, the onset has been indolent and the course progressive (Table 10–1). In the 23 adults, 74% had a steadily progressive course while an additional 17% progressed in a stepwise fashion. In the patients with a progressive course, one had an acute onset whereas in the remainder, symptoms came on insidiously, over a period of many months. Only two adults (9%) had a relapsing course; in both, the onset of the initial episode was acute and they were thought to have GBS until an identical clinical syndrome recurred 2 and 30 months later. One patient had had a severe relapse, necessitating ventilatory support, 2 months after the onset of her initial "GBS," before making a clinically complete recovery after retreatment with plasma exchange. Thirty months later, 2 months after parturition, she relapsed but again spontaneously remitted over a period of months. The other patient had typical GBS that rapidly resolved with plasmapheresis, only to relapse 2 months later. She subsequently ran a remitting–relapsing course. In contrast to the adults, only one of seven children had a progressive course and none was relapsing. The remainder had a monophasic course of weakness that evolved to reach a nadir after 4 to 6 months and then improved slowly. Three children had an acute onset of symptoms and were initially thought to have GBS but their weakness continued to worsen. In these children, follow-up is insufficient to determine whether they will eventually relapse.

The LSU experience contrasts with that reported in the literature.[1–3] In the reported series, the course is progressive in about half of the patients, and

Table 10–1. Characteristics of CIDP in 30 Patients Seen at LSU 1988–1992

	23 ADULTS (%)	7 CHILDREN (%)
Clinical features		
Predominantly sensory	2 (9)	0 (0)
Predominantly motor	13 (57)	3 (43)
Equal sensory and motor	8 (31)	4 (57)
Cranial nerve involvement	0 (0)	5 (71)
Autonomic involvement	1 (4)	1 (14)
Respiratory failure	0 (0)	1 (14)
Asymmetry	9 (39)	0 (0)
Mode of onset		
Acute	3 (13)	3 (43)
Subacute/chronic	20 (87)	4 (57)
Clinical course		
Progressive/stepwise	17/4 (74/17)	1/0 (14/0)
Relapsing	2 (9)	0 (0)
Monophasic	0 (0)	6 (86)
Electrodiagnosis		
Definite demyelination with mild axonal degeneration	13 (57)	6 (86)
Definite demyelination with marked axonal degeneration	9 (39)	0 (0)
Predominantly axonal	1 (4)	1 (14)
Pathology (sural nerve) (9 patients)	5	4
Predominantly demyelinating	3 (60)	4 (100)
Predominantly axonal	2 (40)	0 (0)
Inflammation	4 (80)	1 (25)

progression may be stepwise or inexorable. About 30% to 40% run a relapsing course, with improvement and long periods of stability, sometimes lasting many years. In the small LSU series, as well as some of the reports in the literature, younger patients are more likely to run a relapsing course. Both of our relapsing patients were under 30 years of age and in McCombe et al.'s series the mean age of onset for relapsing patients was 27 years compared to 51 years for progressive patients.[2] The relapsing cases almost invariably eventually accumulate a fixed neurological deficit, in a manner analogous to multiple sclerosis. Occasionally (10–15% of cases) the course is monophasic, with the peak deficit being reached within a period of months before stabilization or improvement occurs. The different experiences with relapse may relate to length of follow-up and to changing patterns of treatment. In the LSU patients, length of follow-up is much shorter, ranging from 9 months to 3 years, and almost all of the patients have received some sort of immunosuppressive treatment that has probably altered the natural history.

Symptoms and Signs

In all of the LSU patients there were both sensory and motor abnormalities. However, in more than half of the entire group (57% of adults and 43% of children) there was a striking predominance of weakness with sensory abnormalities limited to trivial paresthesiae, mild sensory loss in the distal legs, or reduced or absent reflexes. It seems paradoxical that children had a lower proportion of predominantly motor cases since sensory features are more likely to be underplayed in children. Most of the other patients (31% of adults and 57% of children) had approximately equal sensory and motor involvement, although two adults had a marked predominance of sensory symptoms and signs. Weakness is usually accompanied by muscle atrophy, although in some muscles preservation of muscle bulk in the face of significant weakness has provided an important clinical clue to the underlying pathology. All sensory modalities are involved to some extent but proprioception and vibration sense bear the brunt of the sensory loss. Although some reflex loss is invariable in CIDP, it is not as pronounced or as widespread as in GBS, reflecting the more restricted pathology. Cranial nerve involvement is rare in CIDP compared to GBS. None of the adults in the LSU series had cranial neuropathy, although five of the seven children had facial weakness. Autonomic involvement and respiratory failure were also rare. One adult had mild urinary difficulties and one child had evidence of minor sympathetic overactivity. No adult had symptoms of compromised respiratory function but one child developed respiratory failure that required prolonged ventilatory support.

Whereas almost all reports emphasize the symmetry of the neurological deficits in CIDP, we found that some degree of asymmetry was common except in children. Furthermore, in nine of the adults (39%) asymmetry was striking. For example, one man developed first a median and then an ulnar neuropathy in the right arm without signs of overt neuropathy elsewhere. More than a year later he developed pain and numbness in his left hand and both feet and mild foot drop. His electrophysiological studies showed unequivocal demyelination and his neuropathy has responded to treatment with high dose intravenous immunoglobulin. Even when the neuropathy is symmetrical at the time of the initial evaluation, there is often a history of focal or asymmetric onset.

In the LSU series of patients, CIDP bore more of a resemblance to GBS in children than it did in adults. Children tended to have a monophasic, albeit subacute, course. They also had more cranial nerve and respiratory involvement and the pattern of involvement was more symmetrical.

The clinical spectrum of CIDP in the LSU patients differs in several respects from that reported in the literature. Although there is a universal consensus that both sensory and motor functions are involved in almost all patients, motor predominance has been noted in only 10% to 20% of patients reported previously,[1-3] whereas in more than half of our patients it was striking. All are agreed that sensory predominance is rare. Cranial involvement, most commonly facial weakness, has been reported in 15% to 25% of patients, notably more frequent than we have found. Respiratory failure of some degree also appears to be somewhat more common than we have seen but the exact prevalence is uncertain. In the series of Dyck et al.,[1] 11% of patients developed some compromise of respiratory function but it is not clear how severe it was. Autonomic neuropathy appears to be very rare; McCombe et al.[2] found no patient with evidence of autonomic neuropathy whereas Dyck found that 4 of 53 patients were impotent and 2 of 53 were incontinent.[1] Other reports have not mentioned autonomic features and we found few. Asymmetry of the clinical findings has not been commented on previously in large series of cases. In fact, symmetrical involvement is a requirement for diagnosis in some reports[3] and is tacitly assumed in others.[1] The sometimes striking multifocal distribution of the demyelinative lesions has been noted in reports of small numbers of patients. Lewis et al.,[5] in particular, described a group of patients with CIDP evolving with a mononeuropathy multiplex pattern. There was little tendency for the neurological deficit to become bilateral or symmetrical, even after many years. Kinship with CIDP was established by the almost identical electrophysiological and pathological features and a similar, albeit less gratifying, response to treatment. It should not be surprising that a disease in which the pathology is multifocal might sometimes have an overtly multifocal distribution of findings, at least at some stage during its evolution. Bilateral involvement is certainly the rule, as is a tendency to become symmetrical with time, in a manner analogous to the ultimately symmetrical pattern of clinical findings in multiple sclerosis. However, ignorance of the sometimes striking asymmetry may result in misdiagnosis or deprive a patient of potentially effective early treatment or may lead to inappropriate treatment. For example, in the patient described above, the presentation with median and then ulnar neuropathy led to no less than four surgical decompressions before the neuropathy became more generalized and its true nature was recognized.

Various other clinical features have occasionally been found. As with any chronic demyelinating neuropathy, there may be nerve hypertrophy[1,6] that is occasionally dramatic, equaling that seen in the inherited demyelinating neuropathies such as hereditary motor sensory neuropathy, type I (HMSN-I). Spinal cord compression from hypertrophied spinal nerve roots has been reported.[7] When this occurs in young people there is a particular propensity for misdiagnosis and delay of treatment. If there is no family history of a similar disorder in a patient with suspected HMSN-I, careful electrodiagnostic studies and nerve biopsy should be performed before a diagnosis of this untreatable neuropathy is made. For example, we have seen a 38-year-old woman with neuropathy but no family history of neuropathy who carried a diagnosis of HMSN-I primarily because of dramatic nerve hypertrophy. However, her neuropathy was asymmetrical and her nerve conduction studies showed focal temporal dispersion of the compound action muscle potential

(CMAP) and perhaps conduction block. Sural nerve biopsy (Fig. 10–1) showed marked endoneurial edema and onion bulb formation but many myelinated axons were normal and others were only mildly affected. Scattered inflammatory cells were found in the epineurium and one small collection was seen in the subperineurial space of the endoneurium. Despite moderately severe associated axonal degeneration, she responded to treatment with high dose prednisone, plasmapheresis, and the later addition of azathioprine. This case also underscores the importance of electrodiagnosis in distinguishing inherited from acquired demyelinating neuropathies, as will be discussed later.

Tremor is an uncommon feature in CIDP but may occur, particularly in those patients with significant proprioceptive sensory loss.[1,8] Similarly, ataxia and pseudoathetosis are occasionally seen in the same setting.[9] Papilledema occurs in CIDP with about the same frequency that it is seen in GBS. It occurred in 7% of Dyck's patients[1] but was much less common in other series and we have not seen it in our current patients. Central nervous system involvement is more common in CIDP than it is in GBS, as reviewed in Chapter 2, but it is rarely of clinical significance.

Prognosis

Prognosis in CIDP is rather gloomy, at least compared with GBS. Mortality is low in most series, although Dyck et al. attributed death to complications of CIDP in 6 (11%) of their patients.[1] However, few patients recover completely.

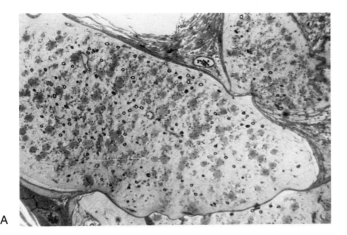

A

Figure 10–1. This sural nerve biopsy was taken from a 38-year-old woman with a slowly progressive sensory motor neuropathy with marked nerve hypertrophy who carried a diagnosis of HMSN-I. She underwent sural nerve biopsy because of clinical and electrophysiological evidence of multifocal peripheral nerve involvement, inconsistent with the initial diagnosis. In **A**, this low power photomicrograph shows both striking endoneurial edema and onion bulb formation, which account for the nerve hypertrophy. (Figure continued on next page)

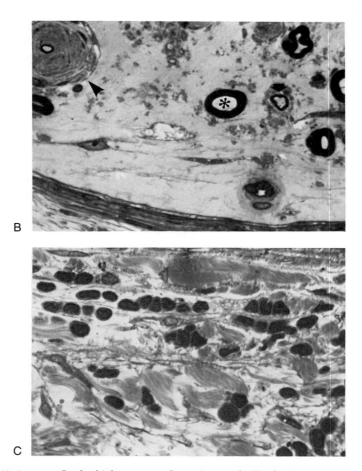

Figure 10–1, cont. In the higher power photomicrograph (**B**), the juxtaposition of normally myelinated axons (*), thinly myelinated axons without onion bulb formation (*arrow*), and advanced onion bulbs (*arrowhead*) within a single high power field identify this as an acquired demyelinating neuropathy rather than HMSN-I. In **C**, a small subperineurial collection of lymphocytes is seen, confirming the inflammatory nature of the demyelinating neuropathy. Treatment with corticosteroids and azathioprine resulted in improvement of the neuropathy.

In Dyck's patients who survived to be evaluated in July 1974, 60% had some neurological problems but remained employed, 8% were still ambulatory but unable to work, 28% were in a wheelchair or confined to bed, and only 4% had recovered. More recent studies paint a less grim picture. For example, McCombe et al.[2] report a mortality of less than 6%, but 73% were independent with only mild functional disability. Perhaps surprisingly, the patients with chronic progressive CIDP fared no worse than those with a relapsing course. Barohn et al.[3] report a mortality of only 3%. We have had no deaths in our patients and all but one remain functional and working with varying degrees of disability, although our follow-up period is much shorter. The most obvious variable in the different series is treatment. In Dyck's patients, 38 of 53 were treated with corticosteroids, in doses ranging from 60 to 80 mg daily, but then tapering and stopping after only 3 to 6 months of treatment. In contrast, McCombe et al.'s patients received steroids for longer periods and steroid failures were treated with other immunosuppressives or with plasmapheresis, with good responses reported in most. Almost all of Barohn et al.'s patients were treated with steroids but the dosage and duration of administration were not noted. We have treated almost all of our patients with high dose intravenous immunoglobulin; a few have received pulsed cyclophosphamide or high dose corticosteroids. Although other variables may have influenced outcome, these cumulative results suggest that treatment does improve the long-term prognosis of the disease.

Epidemiology

CIDP is much less common than GBS and its epidemiology is not so well studied. As with GBS, the disease is more common in men by an almost 2:1 ratio.[1–3] CIDP affects all age groups but the disease frequency increases with age, at least during the first six decades; very few cases with onset over the age of 70 years have been described. Antecedent events are uncommon in most series (10–20%), including our own, although in one study, 32% of patients had had a preceding infection (most commonly cytomegalovirus) or vaccination.[2]

Diseases that are thought to have an autoimmune basis are more often associated with CIDP than one would expect from chance, although the number of reported cases is small. Association with thyrotoxicosis, psoriasis, eczema, urticaria, iritis,[2] Hashimoto's thyroiditis,[10] inflammatory bowel disease, and chronic active hepatitis[3] have been described. One of our patients developed systemic lupus erythematosus more than 5 years after the onset of her neuropathy, an association that has been reported several times.[11–13] An acquired demyelinating neuropathy, virtually indistinguishable from idiopathic CIDP, occurs in association with a variety of abnormalities of serum immunoglobulins but, for the purpose of this discussion, these are considered a separate entity. Unlike GBS, women with CIDP are more likely to develop disease or suffer a relapse during pregnancy or the puerperium.[14,15] In keeping with its probable autoimmune pathogenesis, there is a significant increase in the prevalence of certain histocompatibility antigens, as discussed in Chapter 7. CIDP may also occur in association with human immunodeficiency virus (HIV) infection.[16] It is more common in seropositive patients who are otherwise asymptomatic or in those with minor immune deficiency, such as the lymphadenopathy syndrome or the acquired immunodeficiency syndrome (AIDS)-related complex.[17]

Diagnostic Testing

The clinical features of CIDP are seldom sufficiently characteristic to allow a certain distinction from other chronic neuropathies. Preservation of bulk in weak muscles and disproportionate areflexia are clinical clues to an underlying demyelinating pathology but are unreliable. Therefore, all patients with peripheral neuropathy should have detailed electrodiagnostic studies as a prelude to further investigation. We have found that, in most cases, a confident diagnosis of an acquired demyelinating neuropathy can be made using the electrophysiological studies alone. Nerve biopsy plays a predominantly confirmatory role although occasionally it provides essential diagnostic information unobtainable by other means. Examination of the cerebrospinal fluid is traditionally done but we have found that it adds little useful diagnostic information. There are no specific abnormalities of blood, although it may provide evidence of an associated covert systemic illness.

Electrodiagnostic Studies

As with GBS, the electrodiagnostic studies are the cornerstone on which the accurate and timely diagnosis of CIDP is based. We have found them to be abnormal in all of our patients. In 13 adults and 6 children there was unequivocal electrophysiological evidence of demyelination. Demyelination was also the predominant abnormality in these patients; that is, there was only minor associated axonal degeneration. Another nine adults had definite demyelination in some nerves but with severe associated axonal degeneration. In only two patients (one adult and one child) were there insufficient features to make a confident diagnosis of demyelination on electrophysiological grounds. In both, there was evidence of severe axonal degeneration that made the electrophysiological diagnosis difficult but inflammatory demyelination was found on nerve biopsy. A similar yield of electrodiagnosis was found by Barohn et al.[2]; in their series of 60 patients, 55 had definite evidence of demyelination; 43 had these findings accompanied by significant axonal degeneration. Electrodiagnostic studies are regularly abnormal in other reports, although insufficient details are given to determine the prevalence and extent of abnormalities. It should be stressed that, in keeping with the multifocal distribution of the pathology, conduction may be normal in some nerves and abnormal in others. This is particularly true early in the course of the disease when a strikingly patchy distribution of conduction abnormalities may be seen. Therefore, as in GBS, multiple segments of several nerves should be studied, concentrating on areas of clinical involvement.

    The most common electrodiagnostic abnormality is significant slowing of maximal motor conduction velocity, often into the 15- to 25-m/s range. The patchy distribution of the pathology may be evident not only from side to side but also from nerve to nerve and even from segment to segment within a particular nerve. For example, marked conduction slowing may be seen in the distal segments of motor nerves causing profound prolongation of distal motor latency or severe slowing in the forearm while conduction more proximally remains normal (Fig. 10–2). Compared with GBS, CIDP has less of a predilection for nerve roots so that prolongation of the F-wave latency is usually proportional to the slowing in more peripheral segments. However, in some patients, marked prolongation of F-wave latency in an otherwise pre-dominantly axonal neuropathy may indicate that the primary pathology is demyelination. With time, conduction slowing becomes widespread, usually involving almost all nerves to some extent, although even in advanced cases, slowing is not equal in all areas. In this important respect, CIDP differs from the inherited demyelinating neuropathies in which, from an early age, conduction is slowed to an almost identical degree in all segments of all

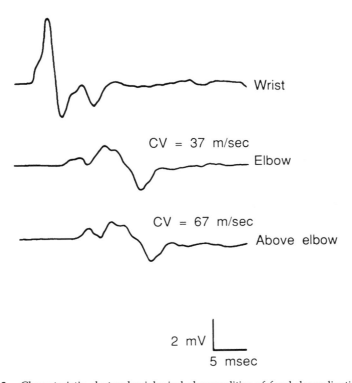

Figure 10–2. Characteristic electrophysiological abnormalities of focal demyelination in the median nerve in a patient with CIDP. The CMAP evoked by stimulation at the wrist (*upper trace*) is of reduced amplitude (4 mV) and is dispersed. With stimulation at the elbow (*middle trace*) there is a 75% fall in the amplitude due to marked temporal dispersion and possibly also conduction block. Distal motor latency is normal but conduction velocity between elbow and wrist is very slow (37 m/s). When the nerve is stimulated in the arm (*lower trace*) there is no further change in the amplitude or waveform and conduction velocity is normal, indicating that changes are focal, confined to the forearm.

nerves.[18,19] Slowing of sensory nerve conduction velocity may also be seen. However, like GBS, some sensory nerves may be relatively spared. Furthermore, when sensory nerves are involved the sensory nerve action potential is usually absent so that conduction slowing cannot be demonstrated. This occurs both because of the associated axon loss and the combination of conduction block and phase cancellation in dispersed sensory responses. Nonetheless, if large numbers of sensory responses are computer averaged to separate the biological signal from background electrical noise, severe conduction slowing in sensory nerves can usually be demonstrated.

The electrodiagnostic abnormalities most specific for CIDP are conduction block and focal dispersion of the CMAP. Conduction block is discussed in detail in Chapter 4 so this discussion will not be reiterated here. Suffice to say that the confident diagnosis of conduction block in chronic neuropathies is more difficult than it is in GBS. From the point of view of identifying focal or multifocal demyelination, the presence of focal dispersion of the CMAP carries as much weight as conduction block and distinguishing between the two is not critical. What is critical is that the change must be shown to be confined to a restricted segment of nerve. CMAP amplitude may fall over a nerve segment such as the forearm segment of the median nerve, due to phase cancellation occurring with a few polyphasic motor units in severely denervated muscles, as discussed in Chapter 4. However, there would be a further fall in amplitude arm segment of the nerve. In CIDP a confident diagnosis rests on the ability to demonstrate that the change in amplitude, negative peak area, and waveform occur over a restricted segment of nerve. For example, if there is a significant change in the waveform of the CMAP between the wrist and elbow in the median nerve but no further change when the nerve is stimulated in the upper arm, then the conduction change, whether it be conduction block or dispersion, has been localized to the forearm segment of that nerve (Fig. 10–2). This localization can be further refined by stimulating the nerve at 5-cm intervals in the forearm, either with surface electrodes or near-nerve needles, so that the length of nerve over which the changes occur can be better defined. In inherited demyelinating neuropathies, chronic axonal neuropathies, and motor neuron diseases the changes in the CMAP occur smoothly, along the entire length of the nerve, and cannot be localized to a restricted nerve segment.

Having established the presence of focal demyelination, it is important, from a prognostic point of view, to assess the extent and severity of the associated axonal degeneration. Significant axonal degeneration almost invariably accompanies the demyelination in CIDP and occasionally it is the predominant abnormality at the time of diagnosis. Electrophysiologically this is manifested as low amplitude or absent sensory and motor responses with denervation of muscles found on needle electromyography (EMG).

There are few substantive differences in the electrophysiological characteristics between GBS and CIDP (Table 10–2). The quintessential features of both are marked conduction slowing, conduction block, differential dispersion, and variable denervation of muscles on needle EMG. GBS has more of a

Table 10–2. Electrophysiological Features of GBS and CIDP

	GBS	CIDP
Diffuse slowing of MCV	+	+ +
More proximal slowing (F-waves)	+ +	+
More distal slowing (DML)	+ +	+
Conduction block	+ + +	+
Differential dispersion	+ +	+ +
Abnormal SNAPs	+	+ + +
Signs of axonal degeneration	+	+ +

+ = uncommon; + + = common; + + + = almost invariable.

predilection for ventral nerve roots so the F-waves are more likely to be absent or have disproportionately prolonged latencies. Similarly, the most distal segments of motor nerves are more often preferentially involved in GBS so the distal motor latencies are prolonged and the distally elicited CMAP dispersed. Conversely, sensory responses are more likely to be abnormal in CIDP, conduction slowing is more widespread, and there is usually a greater degree of associated axonal degeneration. However, none of these differences is absolute and the distinction rests on the temporal profile, not the electrophysiology.

Perhaps the most common cause of misdiagnosis in CIDP is failure to recognize the sometimes predominance of axonal degeneration in this primary demyelinating neuropathy. In many cases, particularly those of long duration, widespread, advanced axonal degeneration prevents recognition of the characteristic electrophysiological changes associated with demyelination. Sensory nerve action potentials (SNAPs) are unobtainable and motor responses are of low amplitude, making it difficult to identify conduction block or differential dispersion. Furthermore, with these low amplitude responses, conduction slowing may be attributed to loss of the largest myelinated axons or to technical factors, or a combination of both. In any patient with a chronic idiopathic neuropathy, particularly if there are signs of overt or covert multifocality, it is important to determine the underlying primary pathology, even if the predominant pathology at the time of evaluation is axonal degeneration. Careful multisegmental studies of several different motor nerves, including measurement of late responses, should be carried out, looking for changes in CMAP amplitude/area, waveform, and conduction velocity that occur over localized segments as well as disproportionate prolongation of F-wave latencies. If the underlying primary pathology remains doubtful, a nerve biopsy should be performed.

Nerve Biopsy

Nerve biopsy is a valuable adjunct in the diagnosis of CIDP, particularly in cases that are electrophysiologically obscure. We performed nerve biopsy in only 9 of our 30 patients, a much lower proportion than usually reported. For example, 87 of 92 patients were biopsied in McCombe et al.'s series[2] and 56 of 60 in Barohn et al.'s.[3] We prefer to place diagnostic emphasis on the electrophysiological studies that have the advantage that many nerves can be sampled over a considerable portion of their length and multiple studies can be performed if the diagnosis is in doubt. We have found that they provide a confident diagnosis in most cases. However, in some cases the degree of associated axonal degeneration or the location of the lesions make a positive electrophysiological diagnosis difficult. This is particularly true when sensory nerve action potentials are absent and the motor responses are of very low amplitude. In such cases, morphological examination of a biopsied nerve (usually the sural) may establish the diagnosis.

The quintessential pathological feature of CIDP is inflammatory demyelination. In seven of nine of our patients who were biopsied, the predominant abnormality was segmental demyelination and remyelination with only mild to moderate axonal degeneration (Fig. 10–3), despite the fact that the SNAP was unobtainable in most, indicating that the absent response was due to dispersion and phase cancellation, not axon loss. There was a variable increase in the number of thinly myelinated axons; occasional axons appeared to be completely devoid of myelin, at least at the light microscopic level. Occasionally, alongside apparently intact demyelinated axons, macrophages containing partly digested myelin could be seen. However, in most cases there was only minimal active myelin degeneration. Hypertrophic changes with rudimentary onion bulb formations were common (Fig. 10–4)

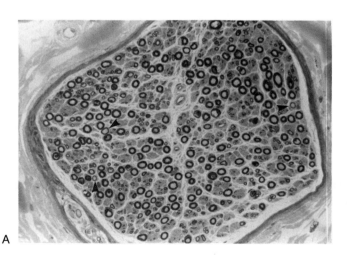

A

Figure 10–3.   This sural nerve biopsy is from a patient with typical CIDP that evolved in a subacute fashion. In **A**, mild endoneurial edema can be seen, concentrated in the subperineurial region and in intrafascicular septae. There is only minimal axon loss and only rare thinly myelinated axons (*arrowheads*). (Figure continued on next page)

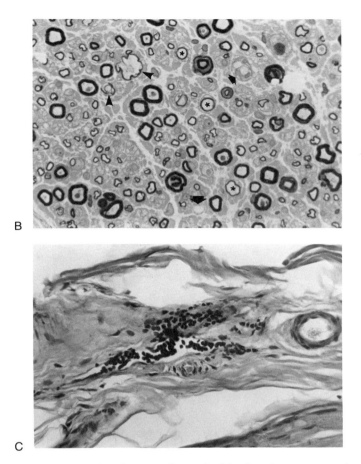

Figure 10–3, cont. In **B**, taken from an adjacent fascicle, there is more severe demyelination. Myelinated axons are at different stages of myelination. In some axons the myelin is in the process of disintegrating and is being peeled away from the underlying axon (*arrowheads*). In others, demyelination is complete without evidence of remyelination, at least at this magnification (*arrows*). Still others have begun to remyelinate but the myelin sheath is still very thin (*). **C** shows a small collection of lymphocytes in the epineurium.

and in a few cases they were well developed (Fig. 10–1). Even when there were marked hypertrophic changes there were important differences from HMSN-I. In CIDP, there was marked variability in the state of myelination from axon to axon within the same fascicle (Fig. 10–1, middle panel). Normally myelinated axons were interspersed with thinly myelinated axons as well as rudimentary and advanced onion bulbs. In contrast, all axons are at approximately the same stage of pathology in HMSN-I; some variability exists but completely normally myelinated axons are never seen juxtaposed against

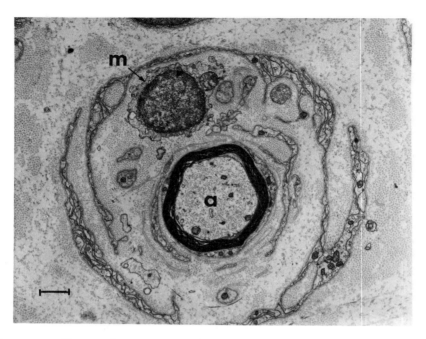

Figure 10–4. Electron photomicrograph of a rudimentary onion bulb formation in a patient with relapsing CIDP. The axon (*a*) is thinly myelinated and is surrounded by redundant Schwann cell processes. A mononuclear cell (*m*) is seen within the Schwann cell processes. (Photomicrograph provided by Dr. John Pollard.)

advanced onion bulbs. Teased fiber preparations confirmed the segmental nature of the demyelination.

In all nine patients there was some axonal degeneration and in two it was severe. However, even in those two patients, those axons that remained showed changes of segmental demyelination with remyelination. Inflammatory changes were seen in four of five adults but only one of four children and the inflammation was also more pronounced in the adults. In all cases it consisted of epineurial perivascular (mainly perivenular) lymphocytic infiltration. Endoneurial inflammation was not seen in the patients in this series, but we have occasionally seen this previously (Fig. 10–1). However, endoneurial edema was common, usually concentrated in the subperineurial space and extending into the fascicle along intrafascicular septae (Fig. 10–3). Severe, diffuse endoneurial edema is occasionally seen (Fig. 10–1). One feature that was commonly seen in our patients was patchy involvement, not only from fascicle to fascicle but even within a single fascicle. This has been alluded to by others and has led to the suggestion that ischemia may play a role in the pathogenesis of the nerve injury in CIDP.[20] However, it may equally reflect a patchy antibody-mediated, inflammatory attack on the nerve.[21]

The changes in our patients are essentially the same as those reported in the literature. However, qualitatively the changes in our patients were more severe, reflecting our selection of cases with severe electrophysiological abnormalities. In all reported series there was segmental demyelination/ remyelination with varying degrees of axonal degeneration. For example, myelinated fiber density was normal in 19 of 26 patients with relapsing CIDP reported by Prineas and McLeod.[22] In most patients with fiber loss, the normal bimodal distribution of fiber diameters is preserved, although there is occasionally preferential loss of large fibers. Dyck et al.[1] found reduced myelinated fiber counts in all of their patients, even those with no clinical sensory abnormalities. Barohn et al.[3] found 18% of biopsies were normal underscoring the disadvantage of nerve biopsy as the sole diagnostic test in this multisegmental disease. Dyck et al.[1] found inflammatory changes in 54% of their biopsies, almost identical to the incidence in our small series (five of nine). However, Barohn et al.[3] found inflammation in only 11% of their biopsies and Oh failed to find inflammation in any of his patients.[23] The reason for such marked differences in the prevalence of inflammation is not immediately apparent. However, inflammation is notoriously patchy and it is possible that insufficient sections were examined in some studies. Inflammation is notably more conspicuous in CIDP related to HIV infection. Endo- neurial edema, which we have found to be common in our more severe cases, has received little attention, although Dyck et al. noted edema in 5 of 26 nerves. A few autopsy studies have been performed and they confirm that the demyelination is widespread but patchy and that it is invariably more widespread than the clinical findings would suggest.

Cerebrospinal Fluid

Although the cerebrospinal fluid (CSF) is often abnormal in CIDP we have not found that CSF examination is diagnostically useful. It simply indicates that the nerve roots are involved in the disease process and is not specific for inflammatory neuropathy. However, elevation of CSF protein may provide an important clue to an otherwise doubtful diagnosis, for example, in cases with advanced axonal degeneration. In the series of Dyck et al.[1] the CSF protein was elevated on at least one occasion in 40 of the 44 patients in whom it was examined. The elevation was usually modest, although values as high as 600 mg/dl were reported. The percentage of gammaglobulin was increased in only six patients, two of whom also had increased serum gammaglobulin. Similarly, Barohn et al.[3] found 95% of their patients had elevated CSF protein. CSF protein is usually more severely elevated in GBS. A modest CSF pleo- cytosis is occasionally found (<10% of cases), although it is the rule in those CIDP patients who are infected with HIV.

Blood

As mentioned, there are no abnormalities of the blood that are of diagnostic utility in idiopathic CIDP. A mild, polyclonal increase in the gammaglobulin fraction of the serum proteins was found in some patients by Dyck et al.[1] A proportion of patients with acquired demyelinating neuropathy will have more specific abnormalities of circulating immunoglobulins (monoclonal gammopathy). We and others[1,2] have excluded these patients from the analysis of CIDP, but Barohn et al.[3] included them. We believe that some minor but consistent differences in clinical presentation, electrophysiology, nerve morphology, and perhaps response to treatment suggest that the paraproteinemic neuropathies may be a distinct entity and we agree with Dyck[24] that they should be treated as such. However, all patients with any chronic idiopathic neuropathy should be carefully screened for immunoglobulin abnormalities.

A routine serum protein electrophoresis will detect most circulating monoclonal proteins although occasionally the monoclonal spike is so small that it is missed.[25] Therefore, sera should be examined by immunoelectrophoresis or immunofixation, at least in those patients whose neuropathy is sufficiently severe to contemplate therapy. Rarely, the monoclonal protein may precipitate as the blood cools while clotting and will be missed entirely if the electrophoresis is done on serum from blood clotted at room temperature. If the index of suspicion is high for a neuropathy associated with monoclonal gammopathy, the electrophoresis should be repeated on blood clotted at 37°C.[26] Circulating monoclonal proteins may be seen in a variety of myeloproliferative diseases such as Waldenstrom's macroglobulinemia, multiple myeloma and solitary plasmacytoma, leukemia, lymphoma, and amyloidosis, although more often no specific associated disease is identified [monoclonal gammopathy of undetermined significance (MGUS)].[27] However, if serum screening identifies a monoclonal protein, a bone marrow examination and a radiographic skeletal survey should be performed to exclude a myeloproliferative disease.

Along the same lines, CIDP may occasionally be associated with a number of other systemic diseases, as discussed in the section on epidemiology, and the blood may provide important clues to a covert systemic disorder. We therefore test for thyroid abnormalities and obtain a complete blood count, antinuclear antibody screen, and sedimentation rate.

Differential Diagnosis

A host of neuropathies resemble CIDP since its clinical features are largely nonspecific. It is for this reason that any patient with a chronic neuropathy should be carefully evaluated with electrophysiological studies and, if necessary, nerve biopsy to establish the presence of multifocal demyelination and inflammation.

PARAPROTEINEMIC NEUROPATHY

As discussed above, the paraproteinemic neuropathies closely resemble CIDP. In fact, Yeung et al.[28] could find no clinical or electrophysiological differences between idiopathic CIDP and any of the paraproteinemic neuropathies, including those with IgM paraproteins reacting with myelin-associated glycoprotein (MAG). The only differences were morphological; none of the paraproteinemic patients had inflammatory infiltrates and patients with IgM paraproteins reacting with MAG have a characteristic decompaction of myelin that is specific for that disorder. In contrast, we have noted a rather consistent pattern of clinical and electrophysiological abnormalities in patients with neuropathy associated with IgM paraproteinemia with antibodies to MAG. In these patients, we have found that the neuropathy is symmetrical and distally accentuated with equal involvement of sensory and motor functions and progression is slow and inexorable. Electrophysiologically, there is a disproportionate prolongation of the distal motor latency in relation to more proximal conduction velocity, to a degree never seen in HMSN-I and rarely in CIDP.[29] Gosselin et al.[30] also noted some minor but consistent differences between CIDP and paraproteinemic neuropathy including a higher frequency of sensory loss and ataxia, and more severe abnormalities of nerve conduction. Nonetheless, the similarity of paraproteinemic neuropathies to CIDP is sufficient that all patients with CIDP should be evaluated for the presence of a monoclonal protein. If one is found, a more detailed evaluation for lymphoproliferative disorders is indicated.

INHERITED DEMYELINATING NEUROPATHIES

As the demyelination in CIDP becomes more and more widespread, its multifocal distribution becomes inapparent and the pathology appears to be clinically diffuse. Such cases may closely resemble inherited demyelinating neuropathies, particularly HMSN-I. Obviously the key to the diagnosis of an inherited neuropathy is the demonstration that other family members are involved. This is usually easy since the inherited demyelinating neuropathies are most often inherited in an autosomal dominant pattern. However, the neuropathy may be oligosymptomatic in other family members so they need to be evaluated objectively with nerve conduction studies that are always abnormal in affected individuals. Even if no other family members are involved, HMSN-I has several characteristics that enable it to be distinguished from CIDP (Table 10–3). First, although both CIDP and HMSN-I both have severe conduction slowing, the distribution of the slowing usually differs. In HMSN-I, there is diffuse slowing, affecting all segments of all nerves to a closely similar degree whereas in CIDP there is marked variability. Second, focal conduction block or differential dispersion never occurs in uncomplicated HMSN-I.[18,19] Third, on nerve biopsy, all axons in HMSN-I are at about the same stage of demyelination whereas in CIDP normal and severely demyelinated axons may be juxtaposed within a fascicle. Of course, significant inflammation only occurs with CIDP, although it is found in only 50% to 60% of cases.

Rarely, patients with a prednisone-responsive neuropathy, suggesting CIDP, have pes cavus and other musculoskeletal deformities more suggestive of HMSN-I and are found to have asymptomatic relatives with a similar

Table 10–3. Distinguishing HMSN-I from CIDP

	HMSN-I	CIDP
Electrophysiology		
Equal proximal and distal conduction slowing	Always	Rarely
Conduction block	Never	Occasionally
Focal dispersion	Never	Common
Morphology		
Endoneurial edema	No	Common
Variable demyelination		
Axon to axon	No	Common
Within fascicles	No	Common
Between fascicles	No	Common
Inflammation	No	Common (50%)

neuropathy.[31,32] The concurrence of these two disorders is more frequent than would be expected from chance and it has been suggested that the presence of an inherited demyelinating neuropathy may predispose the patient to a later immune-mediated attack on their already abnormal nerves. The presence of elevated CSF protein, which is rare in HMSN-I, or any significant change in the tempo of disease should raise the suspicion of CIDP and treatment should be considered.

TOXIC/METABOLIC NEUROPATHIES

Most intoxications and metabolic disorders do not resemble CIDP since they primarily affect axons and are diffuse in their distribution. However, the same metabolic neuropathies, particularly those associated with diabetes and uremia, may have elevated CSF protein, indicating radicular involvement, may be patchy in their distribution, and may have severe slowing of conduction velocity, suggesting associated demyelination. Fortunately, the severity of the neuropathy is usually roughly proportional to the severity of the underlying disorder so it is usually easy to identify. The problem periodically arises whether a diabetic or uremic patient has coincidental CIDP. Unfortunately, there are few reliable means of distinguishing one from another. The clinical features may be almost identical and each may have elevation of CSF protein as well as conduction slowing and variable axon loss with electrodiagnostic testing. The presence of focal conduction block or differential dispersion strongly favors CIDP, although segmental waveform changes, mimicking CIDP, have been described in diabetic neuropathy.[33] Disproportionate prolongation of F-wave latencies or significant demyelinative electrophysiological abnormalities in proximal nerves also favors a diagnosis of CIDP. Morphologically, significant inflammation on nerve biopsy obviously favors CIDP but minor inflammation is nonspecific. It may be necessary, if the severity of the neuropathy justifies it, to treat with plasmapheresis or high dose intravenous immunoglobulin to see if improvement occurs.

Some toxic neuropathies may also superficially resemble CIDP. Hexane inhalation produces massive accumulation of neurofilaments with giant axonal swellings and secondary demyelination. Clinically, there is a strikingly axon length–dependent neuropathy but conduction velocity may be very slow, reflecting the associated demyelination. However, the electrodiagnostic changes are symmetrical and distally accentuated, rather than patchy, and conduction block is not seen. The diagnostic confusion may be compounded by the nerve biopsy, which shows endoneurial edema as well as axonal degeneration and segmental demyelination with onion bulb formation, all features of CIDP. However, there is no inflammation and there are the characteristic giant axonal swellings. Arsenic intoxication may also cause a subacutely progressive polyradiculoneuropathy with high CSF protein.

MULTIFOCAL MOTOR NEUROPATHY

Parry and Clarke have described a pure motor neuropathy that superficially resembles motor neuron disease and that has been designated as multifocal motor neuropathy (MMN).[34] We believe that MMN is simply a predominantly motor variant of CIDP,[35] whereas others hold that it is a distinct nosological entity,[36] a controversy still unresolved. The subject of MMN and the related controversies have been extensively reviewed recently.[35,37]

MMN is characterized clinically by progressive weakness and muscular atrophy, which may be accompanied by cramps and fasciculations and occasionally myokymia. Atrophy may be severe and is nearly always present in some muscles at the time of diagnosis. However, other muscles may have normal bulk despite severe weakness, an important clue in distinguishing MMN from motor neuron disease. In most cases described, the disease began and remained more prominent in the arms. One of the most striking clinical features is the multifocal distribution of the weakness, which can usually be localized within the territory of individual peripheral nerves. Peripheral nerves may be palpably enlarged or enlargement can be seen with magnetic resonance imaging.[38] Although described as a pure motor neuropathy, minor sensory symptoms and signs are often present. Nonetheless, it is still remarkable to see severe weakness, or even complete paralysis, in muscles innervated by a particular peripheral nerve with essentially normal sensory function in the distribution of that same nerve.

The diagnosis of MMN rests on the nerve conduction studies. Affected nerves show severe, or even complete, motor conduction block and yet sensory conduction through the blocked segment is entirely normal (Fig. 10–5). The conduction block is strikingly focal, confined to segments of 3 to 10 cm.[39] Conduction velocity through these segments is severely slowed but is normal elsewhere. The conduction block is remarkably stable, appearing to be unchanged in degree and located in the same region for many years. Electrophysiological support for the contention that MMN and CIDP are one and the same is provided by patients with otherwise typical CIDP with sensory and motor clinical features who, in some nerves, show severe motor

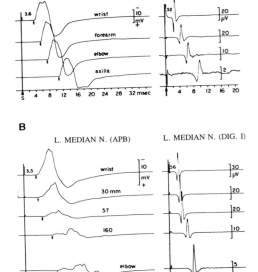

Figure 10–5. Motor and sensory conduction studies of the left median nerve from a control subject (**A**) and a patient with MMN (**B**). The CMAP was recorded from the abductor pollicis brevis (*APB*). The site of stimulation is indicated above the traces (A and B, left column). In the MMN patient, the median nerve was stimulated at the wrist, 30 mm, 57 mm, and 160 mm proximal to the wrist, at the elbow, and at the axilla. The SNAPs evoked by stimulation of digit I were recorded at these same sites. The distal motor latencies and sensory conduction velocities are indicated above the uppermost trace in each column. Despite severe motor conduction block and dispersion of the motor responses in the MMN patient, the decline in the amplitude of the SNAP was not different from the control. (Modified Krarup et al.,[39] with permission.)

block with normal sensory conduction in the same nerve, through the segment of motor block (Fig. 10–6).

Pathologically, MMN is virtually indistinguishable from CIDP, although the changes in biopsied sensory nerves are quantitatively much less severe. Apparently uninvolved sural nerves may show mild segmental demyelination, axon loss, and even lymphocytic inflammation. In one patient, biopsy of a mixed nerve at a site of visible enlargement and corresponding to an area of severe motor conduction block showed chronic demyelination with onion bulb formation but no inflammation.[38]

Patients with MMN may have elevated levels of IgM antibodies to ganglioside, particularly GM1, and some have ascribed a critical pathogenetic role to these antibodies.[36] Although high titers of anti-GM1 antibodies may be seen in MMN, they are occasionally also found in patients with otherwise typical CIDP.[40,41] They also occur in lower titers in patients with motor neuron disease and even in patients with no overt neurological disease. Furthermore, some patients with MMN have normal or only slightly elevated antibody titers. Therefore, the role of these antibodies in the pathogenesis of MMN remains undetermined.

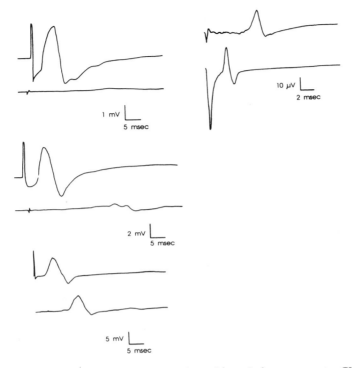

Figure 10–6. Long-term improvement in a patient with typical sensory motor CIDP treated with high dose IVIG. The upper left pair of traces shows a reduced amplitude ulnar CMAP (3.1 mV) with distal stimulation (*upper trace*) with no response with elbow stimulation (*lower trace*), indicating complete conduction block. The upper right tracings are the antidromic sensory responses recorded from the fifth digit with stimulation at the wrist (*lower trace*) and elbow (*upper trace*). These sensory responses are entirely normal, despite complete motor conduction block in the same nerve segment. After a 4-day course of IVIG, the distal ulnar CMAP amplitude has almost doubled to 6.0 mV and a small, dispersed response has appeared with proximal stimulation (*middle traces*). After a further four courses at 3- to 4-month intervals, the ulnar motor nerve conduction has returned to normal (*lower traces*). This patient demonstrates both a dramatic response to IVIG treatment as well as pure motor conduction block in clinically typical sensory motor CIDP.

VASCULITIC NEUROPATHY

Neuropathy may complicate the course of overt systemic necrotizing vasculitis such as polyarteritis nodosa or occasionally be its presenting feature. In such cases, misdiagnosis as CIDP is seldom a problem since the patient has overt systemic disease that usually overshadows the neuropathy. However, a proportion of patients with less malignant, often poorly defined, systemic vasculitides may present with a primarily neuropathic picture. Furthermore, in some cases peripheral nerve appears to be the only organ involved in a vasculitic process.[42,43] These patients may be clinically very similar to CIDP. They have a chronic neuropathy that may evolve in an inexorable or a stepwise progressive fashion. Most patients have overt multifocality (mono-neuropathy multiplex) but in nearly half the multifocality is covert and the neuropathy is simply somewhat asymmetric or may even be completely symmetric. None of these patterns is inconsistent with CIDP. As with CIDP, sensory and motor functions are usually equally involved. In contrast to CIDP, sensory functions subserved by small fibers tend to be more affected. In keeping with greater involvement of small fibers, reflex loss is not as widespread or severe as CIDP.

Electrophysiologically, this neuropathy is characterized by multifocal axonal degeneration. That is, there is loss of amplitude in sensory and motor responses with little slowing of conduction velocity. However, focal changes consistent with conduction block are occasionally seen.[43,44] Needle EMG reveals changes of chronic and ongoing denervation in muscles innervated by affected nerves. The lack of significant conduction slowing is a key to distinguishing CIDP from chronic vasculitic neuropathy. Furthermore, focal conduction block and differential dispersion of motor responses strongly favors a diagnosis of CIDP. Nonetheless, particularly in advanced cases, distinction may be impossible on clinical and electrophysiological grounds and nerve biopsy must be done. Even then the diagnosis may remain in doubt. Necrotizing vasculitis is a patchy process and the biopsy may miss an area of pathognemonic change. The characteristic morphological features of vasculitic neuropathy are multifocal axonal degeneration, rather than de-myelination, with some fascicles involved more than others and with central–fascicular or sector involvement of individual fascicles. Some ischemic de-myelination may be seen but it is usually overshadowed by the axonal degeneration. All of these morphological changes may be seen in patients with CIDP and, unless the changes in the epineurial blood vessels described below are seen, the diagnosis may remain in doubt.

Careful examination of multiple sections from whole nerve, rather than fascicular, biopsy may be necessary to clinch a diagnosis because of the notoriously patchy distribution of the vascular changes. Epineurial blood vessels may be occluded or recanalized, may show fibrinoid necrosis or more often segmental fibrosis of the media, and may have transmural or perivascular inflammatory cells, usually lymphocytes but occasionally, in more acute cases, polymorphonuclear leukocytes. These changes most often involve the arterioles or small arteries, rather than the venules, as is more common in CIDP. Endoneurial inflammation is not seen.

Although not all of the morphological features are seen in every case, the combination of neural and vascular changes usually enables a confident distinction to be made between CIDP and vasculitic neuropathy.

Treatment of CIDP

Although differences exist between CIDP and GBS in their responsiveness to treatment, there are also many similarities. The main difference is in the response to corticosteroid treatment; CIDP has been shown in controlled clinical trials to benefit from steroid treatment whereas GBS does not. However, both disorders appear to respond to plasmapheresis and to high dose intravenous immunoglobulin, although controlled trials establishing the efficacy of the latter in CIDP are lacking.

Corticosteroids

The first detailed report of the efficacy of corticosteroids in CIDP came early, usually in the guise of treatment for GBS; however, many of the cases were clearly relapsing CIDP.[45–48] In 1958, Austin[49] reviewed the subject of "Recurrent polyneuropathies and their corticosteroid treatment" and detailed the results of treatment of 20 episodes of recurrence in a single patient, treated with placebo as well as with several different corticosteroid preparations. This report established without doubt that the patient in question was remarkably steroid responsive. Thereafter, steroids were used widely for the treatment of CIDP and numerous anecdotal reports and uncontrolled studies attested to their efficacy.[8,23,50–52] However, it was not until more than 20 years later that Dyck et al. established, in a controlled trial, that prednisone improved CIDP more than no treatment.[53] They treated 14 patients with CIDP with prednisone for 3 months and 14 closely matched patients received no treatment. They used a tapering dose of prednisone, beginning at 120 mg every other day, reducing each week. They evaluated a number of sensory and motor functions in a semiquantitative manner and found that the treated patients consistently fared better. Although the treatment was effective, the duration of treatment was brief and we have found that much longer periods of treatment are usually needed if the benefit is to be maintained. In addition, it is difficult to taper the steroid dose to a level where adverse effects are acceptable. Thus, although treatment with corticosteroids is frequently beneficial, the chronic nature of the neuropathy usually requires long-term treatment at high doses with the inevitable attendant adverse effects. As a result, alternative treatments with greater efficacy or fewer adverse effects are still being sought.

Plasmapheresis

In 1979, concerned with the risks of steroid treatment in CIDP and encouraged by the reports of response of myasthenia gravis to plasma exchange, Server et al.[54] treated a man with relapsing CIDP with plasmapheresis and noted dramatic improvement with each treatment. Several other reports of efficacy soon followed.[55–60] In 1986, Dyck et al. randomly assigned patients with CIDP to plasma exchange or sham exchange and found that a subset of patients showed a significant improvement.[61] Their subsequent experiences have led them to endorse enthusiastically the frequent use of plasmapheresis in all patients with CIDP in whom the severity of the neuropathy is sufficient to warrant treatment (Dyck, *personal communication*). Long-term use of plasmapheresis over nearly a decade, to maintain function in CIDP patients, has been shown to be both safe and effective, at least in children.[62] More recently, plasmapheresis has been shown also to benefit patients with neuropathy associated with monoclonal gammopathy of undetermined significance, although the benefits were not as encouraging.[63] Our own experiences with plasmapheresis have not been so encouraging and we have largely abandoned it for what we believe to be more effective and better tolerated therapy, namely high dose intravenous immunoglobulin.

Intravenous Immunoglobulin

High dose intravenous immunoglobulin (IVIG) has been widely used for the treatment of many autoimmune disorders.[64] The use of IVIG to treat GBS has been discussed in Chapter 6. There has also been a plethora of reports of the use of IVIG in CIDP. As early as 1981, Maas et al.[65] reported a patient who responded equally well to both plasmapheresis and to infusion of fresh frozen plasma. This same group extended their observations to 17 patients, which they reported in 1985.[66] Thirteen improved and, although the effect was short-lived, they all responded to further infusions. Several more enthusiastic case reports and uncontrolled studies soon followed in patients with idiopathic CIDP,[67,68] HIV-related CIDP,[69] and paraproteinemic neuropathy.[70] One double-blind, placebo-controlled, crossover study has confirmed the efficacy in small numbers of patients.[71] More recently, several investigators have found that IVIG was also effective in patients with multifocal motor neuropathy.[72,73] Results of larger controlled studies are awaited with interest. Our own experience is that some response to treatment is almost invariable, although patients with advanced axonal degeneration, not surprisingly, respond poorly. The response in children has been particularly gratifying, with all but one showing dramatic improvement.[74] Improvement in some cases correlates with increased nerve conduction velocities, increased CMAP amplitudes, and partial reversal of conduction block.[75] We have seen one patient in whom there was rapid partial reversal of conduction block that paralleled clinical improvement after each of several courses of treatment (Fig. 10–7). In some cases, improvement is sustained for many months and we have seen occasional cases in which permanent, or at least very long-lasting, remission has coincided with one or two courses of IVIG. However, in most cases the improvement is short-lived, lasting from 2 weeks to 3 months (Fig. 10–8). Nonetheless, patients appear to retain their responsiveness to the treatment despite many courses and patients have received more than 50 courses without decline in efficacy or adverse effects.

Other Immunosuppressives

There have been no controlled studies of the efficacy of any of the other immunosuppressives as the only treatment. A number of case reports or

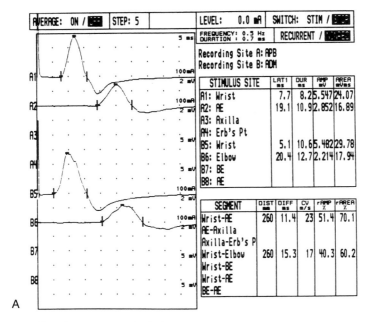

AVERAGE: ON / ▓▓	STEP: 5		LEVEL: 0.0 mA	SWITCH: STIM / ▓▓

FREQUENCY: 0.3 Hz
DURATION : 0.7 ms   RECURRENT / ▓▓▓

Recording Site A: APB
Recording Site B: ADM

STIMULUS SITE	LAT1 ms	DUR ms	AMP mV	AREA mVms
A1: Wrist	7.7	8.2	5.547	24.07
A2: AE	19.1	10.9	2.852	16.89
A3: Axilla				
A4: Erb's Pt				
B5: Wrist	5.1	10.6	5.482	29.78
B6: Elbow	20.4	12.7	2.214	17.94
B7: BE				
B8: AE				

SEGMENT	DIST mm	DIFF ms	CV m/s	rAMP %	rAREA %
Wrist-AE	260	11.4	23	51.4	70.1
AE-Axilla					
Axilla-Erb's P					
Wrist-Elbow	260	15.3	17	40.3	60.2
Wrist-BE					
Wrist-AE					
BE-AE					

Figure 10–7. Rapid response to high dose IVIG therapy in CIDP. The upper panel shows median and ulnar motor nerve conduction studies performed 2 days before IVIG therapy, at a time when the patient was experiencing increasing weakness. In both nerves, there is a significant drop in amplitude of the CMAP between wrist and elbow, suggestive of conduction block. The lower panel shows the same studies repeated 1 day after completing a 4-day course of IVIG. In both nerves, there has been a 20% increase in the proximal CMAP amplitude. The distal CMAP amplitude has also increased slightly, perhaps due to reversal of distal conduction block, but there has been no change in conduction velocity. This same pattern of improvement was seen after each of several courses of treatment.

small, uncontrolled series noted improvement in patients treated with aza-thioprine, usually after prednisone had failed or could not be tolerated.[76–78] However, Dyck et al., in a study of prednisone alone or in combination with azathioprine, found no advantage to the combination.[79] Cyclophosphamide has also been reported to be effective. Several of the GBS patients described by Rosen and Vastola clearly had CIDP and good responses to pulsed intravenous cyclophosphamide were reported.[80] Fowler et al. also reported good response to oral cyclophosphamide but the patient also received con-comitant plasmapheresis.[55] We have found that pulsed cyclophosphamide, administered in a manner similar to that used in the treatment of progressive multiple sclerosis,[81] appears to have induced remission in some patients and is well tolerated but our observations, like those reported in the literature, are completely uncontrolled. CIDP has also been treated with cyclosporin A in three patients who had not responded to steroids, azathioprine, or plasma-pheresis. All improved and one went into complete remission.[82]

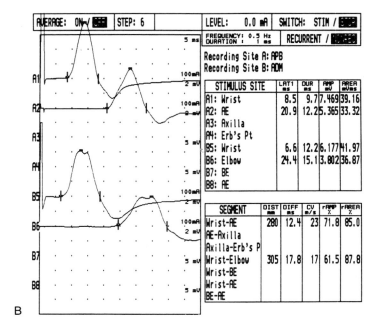

Figure 10–7, cont

From the foregoing it appears that a proportion of patients benefit from a variety of immunosuppressives, although controlled studies are lacking. Given the progressive nature of the disease in most patients and the very low rate of spontaneous remission, it is reasonable that patients who have failed to respond to better proven (corticosteroids, plasmapheresis) or safer (IVIG) treatments should be given a trial of immunosuppressive treatment. The drug of choice and the mode of administration remain the subjects of considerable discussion and no consensus has been reached. We have found that pulsed intravenous therapy is uniformly better tolerated than chronic oral administration, at least for cyclophosphamide, and it may also be more effective.

Summary

Despite a steadily increasing awareness of CIDP, it still remains one of the most underdiagnosed neuropathies. The frequent delay in reaching this diagnosis may have unfortunate consequences, since treatment is clearly most effective if applied early, before significant axonal degeneration has supervened. All chronic neuropathies for which no etiology is immediately forthcoming should be carefully evaluated by means of electrodiagnostic

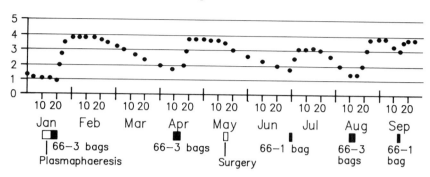

Figure 10–8. Clinical response to repeated courses of IVIG in a patient with CIDP. The vertical axis shows a semiquantitative cumulative strength scale, with 5 being normal, and the horizontal axis shows time. After each treatment, there is a rapid improvement in strength that plateaus for about a month and then slowly deteriorates.

studies by a sophisticated and experienced electromyographer for evidence of segmental demyelination. If questions remain, a nerve biopsy should be done. In this way a timely diagnosis should be reached so that appropriate treatment can be administered while there is still the potential for recovery or at least improvement. The development of safer, and hopefully more effective, therapies will make early diagnosis even more imperative.

References

1. Dyck PJ, Lais AC, Ohta M, Bastron JA, Okazaki H, Groover RV. Chronic inflammatory polyradiculoneuropathy. *Mayo Clin Proc.* 1975;50:621–637.
2. McCombe PA, Pollard JD, McLeod JG. Chronic inflammatory demyelinating polyradiculo-neuropathy. A clinical and electrophysiological study of 92 cases. *Brain.* 1987;110:1617–1630.
3. Barohn RJ, Kissel JT, Warmolts JR, Mendell JR. Chronic inflammatory demyelinating polyradiculoneuropathy. Clinical characteristics, course, and recommendations for diagnostic criteria. *Arch Neurol.* 1989;46:878–884.
4. AIDS Task Force. Research criteria for diagnosis of chronic inflammatory demyelinating polyneuropathy (CIDP). *Neurology.* 1991;41:617–618.
5. Lewis RA, Sumner AJ, Brown MJ, Asbury AK. Multifocal demyelinating neuropathy with persistent conduction block. *Neurology.* 1982;32:958.
6. Austin JH. Observations on the syndrome of hypertrophic neuritis (the hypertrophic interstitial radiculoneuropathies). *Medicine.* 1956;35:187–237.
7. Symons CP, Blackwood W. Spinal cord compression in hypertrophic neuritis. *Brain.* 1962;85:251–259.
8. Dalakas MC, Engel WK. Chronic relapsing (dysimmune) polyneuropathy: pathogenesis and treatment. *Ann Neurol.* 1981;9(suppl):134–145.
9. Dalakas MC. Chronic idiopathic ataxic neuropathy. *Ann Neurol.* 1986;19:545–554.
10. Potz G, Neundorfer B. Polyradicular neuritis and Hashimoto's thyroiditis. *J Neurol.* 1975; 210:283–289.
11. Scheinberg L. Polyneuritis in systemic lupus erythematosus: review of the literature and report of a case. *N Engl J Med.* 1956;255:416–421.

12. Goldberg M, Chitanandh H. Polyneuritis with albuminocytologic dissociation in the spinal fluid in systemic lupus erythematosus. Report of a case with review of pertinent literature. *Am J Med*. 1959;27:342–350.
13. Rechtand E, Cornblath DR, Stern BJ, Meyerhoff JO. Chronic demyelinating polyneuropathy in systemic lupus erythematosus. *Neurology*. 1984;34:1375–1377.
14. McCombe PA, McManis PG, Frith JA, Pollard JD, McLeod JG. Chronic inflammatory demyelinating polyradiculoneuropathy associated with pregnancy. *Ann Neurol*. 1987;21: 102–104.
15. Parry GJ, Heiman-Patterson TD. Pregnancy and autoimmune neuromuscular disease. *Semin Neurol*. 1988;8:197–204.
16. Cornblath DR, McArthur JC, Kennedy PGE, Witte AS, Griffin JW. Inflammatory demyelinating peripheral neuropathies associated with human T-cell lymphotropic virus type III infection. *Ann Neurol*. 1987;21:32–40.
17. Parry GJ. Peripheral neuropathies associated with human immunodeficiency virus infection. *Ann Neurol*. 1988;23(suppl):S49–53.
18. Lewis RA, Sumner AJ. The electrodiagnostic distinctions between chronic familial and acquired demyelinative neuropathies. *Neurology*. 1982;32:592.
19. Parry GJG, Malamut R, Lupski JR, Patel PI, Garcia CA. Nerve conduction studies in hereditary motor and sensory neuropathy, Type I. *Muscle Nerve*. 1991;14:891.
20. Nukada H, Pollock M, Haas LF. Is ischemia implicated in chronic multifocal demyelinating neuropathy? *Neurology*. 1989;39:106–110.
21. Bradley WG. Chronic demyelinating neuropathy. *Neurology*. 1989;39:1270.
22. Prineas JW, McLeod JG. Chronic relapsing polyneuritis. *J Neurol Sci*. 1976;27:427-458.
23. Oh SJ. Subacute demyelinating polyneuropathy responding to corticosteroid treatment. *Arch Neurol*. 1978;35:509–516.
24. Dyck PJ. Intravenous immunoglobulin in chronic inflammatory demyelinating polyradiculoneuropathy and with neuropathy associated with IgM monoclonal gammopathy of unknown significance. *Neurology*. 1990;40:327–328.
25. Kelly JJ. Peripheral neuropathies associated with monoclonal proteins: a clinical review. *Muscle Nerve*. 1985;8:138–150.
26. Sherman WH, Osserman EF, Latov N, Olarte MR, Rowland LP. Peripheral neuropathy, plasma dyscrasia, and hot blood. *Ann Neurol*. 1982;12:319.
27. Kelly JJ, Kyle RA, Latov N. *Polyneuropathies associated with plasma cell dyscrasias*. Boston: Martinus Nijhoff; 1987.
28. Yeung KB, Thomas PK, King RHM, et al. The clinical spectrum of peripheral neuropathies associated with benign monoclonal IgM, IgG and IgA paraproteinemia. Comparative clinical, immunological and nerve biopsy findings. *J Neurol*. 1991;238:383–391.
29. Kaku DA, Sumner AJ. Characteristic electrophysiological findings in anti-MAG polyneuropathy. *Neurology*. 1992;42(suppl3):408. Abstract.
30. Gosselin S, Kyle RA, Dyck PJ. Neuropathy associated with monoclonal gammopathies of undetermined significance. *Ann Neurol*. 1991;30:54–61.
31. Dyck PJ, Swanson CJ, Low PA, Bartleson JD, Lambert EH. Prednisone-responsive hereditary motor and sensory neuropathy. *Mayo Clin Proc*. 1982;57:239–246.
32. Mitchel GW, Bosch EP, Hart MN. Response to immunosuppressive therapy in patients with hereditary motor and sensory neuropathy and associated dysimmune neuromuscular disorders. *Eur Neurol*. 1987;27:188–196.
33. Abu-Shakra SR, Cornblath DR, Avila OL, et al. Conduction block in diabetic neuropathy. *Muscle Nerve*. 1991;14:858–862.
34. Parry GJ, Clarke S. Multifocal acquired demyelinating neuropathy masquerading as motor neuron disease. *Muscle Nerve*. 1988;11:103–107.
35. Parry GJ, Sumner AJ. Multifocal motor neuropathy. *Neurol Clin*. 1992;10:671–684.
36. Pestronk A. Motor neuropathies, motor neuron disorders, and antiglycolipid antibodies. *Muscle Nerve*. 1991;14:927–936.
37. Parry GJ. Motor neuropathy with multifocal conduction block. In: Peripheral Neuropathy. Dyck PJ, Thomas PK, Lambert EH, Griffin J, Low PA, Poduslo J, eds. Philadelphia: Saunders. In press.
38. Kaji R, Oka N, Tsuji T, Mezaki T, Kimura J. Pathological findings at the sites of conduction block in multifocal motor neuropathy. *Ann Neurol*. In press.
39. Krarup C, Stewart JD, Sumner AJ, Pestronk A, Lipton SA. A syndrome of asymmetric limb weakness with motor conduction block. *Neurology*. 1990;40:118–127.

40. Lamb NL, Patten BM. Clinical correlations of anti-GM1 antibodies in amyotrophic lateral sclerosis and neuropathies. *Muscle Nerve.* 1991;14:1021–1027.
41. Sindern E, Stark E, Haas AJ, Steck AJ. Serum antibodies to GM1 and GM3-gangliosides in systemic lupus erythematosus with chronic inflammatory demyelinating polyradiculoneuropathy. *Acta Neurol Scand.* 1991;83:399–402.
42. Kissel JT, Slivka AP, Warmolts JR, Mendell JR. The clinical spectrum of necrotizing angiopathy of the peripheral nervous system. *Ann Neurol.* 1985;18:251–257.
43. Dyck PJ, Benstead TJ, Conn DL, Stevens JC, Windebank AJ, Low PA. Nonsystemic vasculitic neuropathy. *Brain.* 1987;110:843–854.
44. Jamieson PW, Giuliani MJ, Martinez AJ. Necrotizing angiopathy presenting with multifocal conduction blocks. *Neurology.* 1991;41:442–444.
45. Stillman WF, Ganong WF. The Guillain-Barré syndrome: report of a case treated with ACTH and cortisone. *N Engl J Med.* 1952;246:293.
46. Newey JA, Lubin RI. Corticotrophin (ACTH) therapy in Guillain-Barré syndrome. *JAMA.* 1953;152:137–139.
47. Blood A, Locke W, Carabasi R. Guillain-Barré syndrome treated with corticotrophin (ACTH). *JAMA.* 1953;152:139.
48. Plum F. Multiple symmetrical polyneuropathy treated with cortisone. *Neurology.* 1953;3: 661–667.
49. Austin JH. Recurrent polyneuropathies and their corticosteroid treatment. With five-year observations of a placebo-controlled case treated with corticotrophin, cortisone, and prednisone. *Brain.* 1958;81:157–195.
50. Matthews WB, Howell DA, Hughes RC. Relapsing corticosteroid-dependent polyneuritis. *J Neurol Neurosurg Psychiatry.* 1970;33:330–337.
51. DeVivo DC, Engel WK. Remarkable recovery of a steroid-responsive recurrent polyneuropathy. *J Neurol Neurosurg Psychiatry.* 1970;33:62–69.
52. Schwartzman, Engel WK, Rapoport A. Criteria for the prednisone treatment of idiopathic polyneuropathy. *Neurology.* 1977;27:364.
53. Dyck PJ, O'Brien PC, Oviatt KF, et al. Prednisone improves chronic inflammatory polyradiculoneuropathy more than no treatment. *Ann Neurol.* 1982;11:136–141.
54. Server AC, Lefkowith J, Braine H, McKhann GM. Treatment of chronic relapsing inflammatory polyradiculoneuropathy by plasma exchange. *Ann Neurol.* 1979;6:258–261.
55. Fowler H, Vulpe M, Marks G, Egolf C, Dau PC. Recovery from chronic progressive polyneuropathy after treatment with plasma exchange and cyclophosphamide. *Lancet.* 1979;2:1193.
56. Levy RL, Newkirk R, Ochoa J. Treating chronic relapsing Guillain-Barré syndrome by plasma exchange. *Lancet.* 1979;2:259–260.
57. van Nunen SA, Gatenby PA, Pollard JD, Deacon M, Clancy RL. Specificity of plasmapheresis in the treatment of chronic relapsing polyneuropathy. *Aust NZ J Med.* 1982;12:81–84.
58. Gross MLP, Thomas PK. The treatment of chronic relapsing and chronic progressive idiopathic inflammatory polyneuropathy by plasma exchange. *J Neurol Sci.* 1981;52:69–78.
59. Toyka KV, Augspach R, Wietholter H, et al. Plasma exchange in chronic inflammatory polyneuropathy: evidence suggestive of a pathogenic humoral factor. *Muscle Nerve.* 1982;5:479–484.
60. Donofrio PD, Tandan R, Albers JW. Plasma exchange in chronic inflammatory demyelinating polyradiculoneuropathy. *Muscle Nerve.* 1985;8:321–327.
61. Dyck PJ, Daube J, O'Brien P, et al. Plasma exchange in chronic inflammatory polyradiculoneuropathy. *N Engl J Med.* 1986;314:461–465.
62. Beydoun SR, Engel WK, Karofsky P, Schwartz MU. Long-term plasmapheresis therapy is effective and safe in children with chronic relapsing dysimmune neuropathy. *Rev Neurol.* 1990;146:123–127.
63. Dyck PJ, Low PA, Windebank AJ, et al. Plasma exchange in polyneuropathy associated with monoclonal gammopathy of undetermined significance. *N Engl J Med.* 1991;325:1482–1486.
64. Etziono A, Pollack S. High dose intravenous gammaglobulins in autoimmune disorders: mode of action and therapeutic uses. *Autoimmunology.* 1989;3:307–315.
65. Maas AIR, Busch HFM, van der Heul. Plasma infusion and plasma exchange in chronic idiopathic polyneuropathy. *N Engl J Med.* 1981;305:344.
66. Vermeulen M, van der Meche FGA, Speelman JD, Weber A, Busch HFM. Plasma and gamma-globulin infusion in chronic inflammatory polyneuropathy. *J Neurol Sci.* 1985;70: 317–326.

67. Curro Dossi B, Tezzon F. High-dose intravenous gammaglobulin for chronic inflammatory demyelinating polyneuropathy. *Ital J Neurol Sci.* 1987;8:321–326.
68. Faed JM, Day B, Pollock M, Taylor PK, Nukada H, Hammond-Tooke GD. High-dose intravenous immunoglobulin in chronic inflammatory demyelinating polyneuropathy. *Neurology.* 1989;39:422–425.
69. Chimowitz MI, Audet A-MJ, Hallet A, Kelly JJ. HIV-associated CIDP. *Muscle Nerve.* 1989;12:695–696.
70. Cook D, Dalakas M, Galdi A, Biondi D, Porter H. High-dose intravenous immunoglobulin in the treatment of demyelinating neuropathy associated with monoclonal gammopathy. *Neurology.* 1990;40:212–214.
71. van Doorn PA, Brand A, Strengers PFW, Meulstee J, Vermeulen M. High-dose intravenous immunoglobulin treatment in chronic inflammatory demyelinating polyneuropathy: a double-blind, placebo-controlled, crossover study. *Neurology.* 1990;40:209–212.
72. Kaji R, Shibasaki H, Kimura J. Multifocal demyelinating motor neuropathy: cranial nerve involvement and immunoglobulin therapy. *Neurology.* 1992;42:506–509.
73. Chaudry V, Corse AM, Griffin JW, et al. Multifocal motor neuropathy with anti-GM1 antibodies and partial motor conduction block: favorable response to intravenous immunoglobulin therapy. *Neurology.* 1992;42(suppl 3):178. Abstract.
74. Teasley JE, Parry GJ, Sumner AJ. Chronic inflammatory demyelinating polyradiculoneuropathy in children treated with intravenous immunoglobulin. *Muscle Nerve.* 1991;14:921.
75. van der Meche FGA, Vermeulen M, Busch HFM. Chronic inflammatory demyelinating polyneuropathy. Conduction failure before and during immunoglobulin or plasma therapy. *Brain.* 1989;112:1563–1571.
76. Yuill GM, Swinburn WR, Liversedge LA. Treatment of polyneuropathy with azathioprine. *Lancet.* 1970;2:854–856.
77. Walker GL. Progressive polyradiculoneuropathy: treatment with azathioprine. *Aust NZ J Med.* 1979;9:184–187.
78. Pentland B, Adams GGW, Mawdsley C. Chronic idiopathic polyneuropathy treated with azathioprine. *J Neurol Neurosurg Psychiatry.* 1982;45:866–869.
79. Dyck PJ, O'Brien P, Swanson C, Low P, Daube J. Combined azathioprine and prednisone in chronic inflammatory demyelinating polyneuropathy. *Neurology.* 1985;35:1173–1176.
80. Rosen AD, Vastola EF. Clinical effects of cyclophosphamide in Guillain-Barré polyneuritis. *J Neurol Sci.* 1976;30:179–187.
81. Weiner HL, Hafler DA. Immunotherapy of multiple sclerosis. *Ann Neurol.* 1988;23:211–222.
82. Hodgkinson SJ, Pollard LD, McLeod JG. Cyclosporin A in the treatment of chronic demyelinating polyradiculoneuropathy. *J Neurol Neurosurg Psychiatry.* 1990;53:327–330.

Index

Italics indicate a Table or Figure

195

12/2